The Pittsburgh Way to Efficient Healthcare

The Pittsburgh Way to Efficient Healthcare

Improving Patient Care Using Toyota-Based Methods

NAIDA GRUNDEN

Healthcare Performance Press
A Division of Productivity Press

Healthcare Performance Press is a division of Productivity Press.

Most Healthcare Performance Press books are available at quantity discounts when purchased in bulk. For more information, contact our Customer Service Department (888-319-5852). Address all other inquiries to:

Productivity Press
444 Park Avenue South, 7th Floor
New York, NY 10016
United States of America
Telephone: 212-686-5900
Fax: 212-686-5411
E-mail: info@productivitypress.com
HCPpress.com

Library of Congress Cataloging-in-Publication Data
Grunden, Naida.
The Pittsburgh way to efficient healthcare : improving patient care using Toyota-based methods / Naida Grunden.
p. cm.
Comprises stories written over the past six years for the monthly newsletters of the Pittsburgh Regional Health Initiative (PRHI).
Includes bibliographical references and index.
ISBN 978-1-56327-367-4 (alk. paper)
1. Hospital care—Standards—United States. 2. Hospital care—United States—Quality control. 3. Medical errors—United States—Prevention.
I. Pittsburgh Regional Health Initiative. II. Title.
[DNLM: 1. Hospitals—standards—United States—Collected Works.
2. Quality Assurance, Health Care—United States—Collected Works.
3. Cross Infection—prevention & control—United States—Collected Works.
4. Medical Errors—prevention & control—United States—Collected Works.
WX 153 G889p2008]
RA981.A2G78 2008
362.11068—dc22

2007042982

CONTENTS

FOREWORD: THE PITTSBURGH WAY

The healthcare system in the United States is neither a system nor is it designed to promote health. Rather, as astute observers recognize, the whole collective remains expensive, wasteful, and even harmful to tens of thousands of patients each year. Only in the last six years have we recognized the need for a better way. Healthcare leaders around the nation have reached out to industry and have imported tools such as the Toyota Production System and transformed it into a scientific process called Perfecting Patient Care℠.

Yet the Toyota-based discipline of Perfecting Patient Care, which itself relies on observation, standardization, testing, and data has not yet had the conceptual breakthrough it needs to become our new guiding principle. Enter now Naida Grunden and her book *The Pittsburgh Way to Efficient Healthcare*. The question is can *The Pittsburgh Way* become synonymous with the Toyota Way as it applies to improving the quality and safety of medical care in our country?

Neophytes to the movement will likely question the title of this new book. Proponents of the lean manufacturing methodology will shudder at some of the healthcare analogies. Finally, those naysayers committed to a defense of the status quo will simply reject *The Pittsburgh Way* out of hand.

It is my view that this book is just exactly what the doctor ordered—a sort of final bridging document that takes us from lean manufacturing to Perfecting Patient Care in one smooth and efficient journey. We recognize variation and waste in the healthcare system as the true enemies and while we are *not* building cars while we care for patients, we must recognize that measurement, observation, standardization, testing, and data are indeed the roadside markings on that smooth journey to safety and positive outcomes.

Naida Grunden has done it! She has taken the amazing work done by her colleagues at the Pittsburgh Regional Health Initiative (PRHI) and translated it for a broader audience, an audience that will recognize the power of this book to deliver what I envision to be the definitive map on our journey toward quality and safety. Grunden skillfully recognizes that this new way of patient care will also mean perfecting an innovative cultural reality in medicine and overcoming significant cultural barriers related to the training of healthcare professionals. Nurse navigators, the custodial staff, ICU leadership, and hospital presidents are examined in the same light—a light that enables all members of the healthcare team to participate in the journey toward quality and safety. This light illuminates its intense beam on cultural barriers and seeks to destroy them, as though wielding a laser gun.

Who should read this book? This book should be read by everyone, up and down the line, involved in improving the quality and safety of patient care in our country. This book will enlighten classroom conversation in schools of medicine, nursing, public health, and health administration. This book will better inform the debate regarding the road toward quality and safety while it paves the way for a much broader understanding of the concepts behind Perfecting Patient Care.

Grunden brings to life the human element of her cases with clarity of prose and a minimum of jargon. She cuts to the chase with a matter-of-fact style that belies all of the organizational changes that occurred within the PRHI Program. One day in the future, we will look back at *The Pittsburgh Way* as the *only* way to deliver the kind of healthcare we all want for our children and our children's children. Kudos to Grunden and Godspeed to the many well-deserving practitioners who made PRHI possible!

David B. Nash, MD, MBA
May 16, 2007

ACKNOWLEDGMENTS

This book comprises stories I have written over the past six years for the monthly newsletters of the Pittsburgh Regional Health Initiative (PRHI), an organization within the Jewish Healthcare Foundation (JHF) of Pittsburgh. I thank JHF and PRHI for licensing my use of the stories presented in this book, and permitting me to use their service mark, "Perfecting Patient Care." I extend special thanks to Karen Wolk Feinstein, PhD, President of JHF and CEO of PRHI, under whose leadership this work took place. I am also grateful to the Henry Ford Health System, which consented to my use of their story in Section 2 of Chapter 8.

I especially thank Diane Lares Frndak and daughters, Karen and Kristen Lares, for allowing me to tell their story as the frame for this book.

Thanks to Debra Thompson, MSN, RN, who helped design the programs described in Chapter 3, in Section 3 of Chapter 7, Section 2 of Chapter 8, and Section 5 of Chapter 6. And for their thoughtful manuscript review and writing contributions in Chapter 7, thanks to Tania Lyon, PhD, and Pamela Gaynor.

Of course I thank every frontline worker I've interviewed over the past six years—doctors, nurses, pharmacists, technicians, dieticians, housekeepers, and others—and those healthcare industry leaders who let me tell their stories. Frontline workers toil on the sharp end of change, which, in healthcare, is particularly difficult work. The institutions have been brave as well, for acknowledging improvement means acknowledging that things haven't been going perfectly in the first place. In the beginning, admitting to any kind of institutional imperfection meant going out on a limb. The sustained participation of these institutions confirms what medical people of good will already know: that only in revealing problems can they ever be fixed.

Thanks to the people at Healthcare Performance Press, who believed in this project and encouraged me, and to Pamela Gaynor, Tania Lyon and Mimi Falbo for being my mentors.

PREFACE

If you follow the national discussion on patient safety, you've probably read about the work transpiring in Pittsburgh. You may have heard about the Pittsburgh Regional Health Initiative (PRHI), a consortium of business and healthcare leaders that began leading the way toward healthcare improvement a decade ago—long before patient safety became a *cause célèbre*. You may even have read about PRHI's approach to improvements, based on the Toyota Production System, which it refers to as Perfecting Patient Care. Hundreds of people have arranged field trips to various Pittsburgh hospitals and clinics, hoping to catch a glimpse of these improvements in action.

This book is intended as a field guide to the healthcare improvement work begun by PRHI and continued by institutions and practitioners across the Pittsburgh region and beyond. After a brief description of PRHI's early history and its organizational trials and triumphs, each section focuses on a critical area of healthcare, with actual examples of how improvement was achieved on the ground, in real life.

This is not a cookbook, and the improvement stories are not recipes. Instead, they describe specific problems, attempts to solve them, and outcomes that resulted at that place and time. Like the Toyota-based discipline on which it is based, Perfecting Patient Care relies on observation, standardization, testing, and data. People often mistake this approach for regimentation, where one size fits all, but nothing could be further from the truth. By standardizing the work, each institution, each unit, and each worker can see what's working and what isn't, and quickly adjust procedures accordingly. This approach, while disciplined, is almost infinitely adaptable.

Other books and articles describe the nuts and bolts of the Toyota Production System, on which Perfecting Patient Care is based.[1,2,3,4] This book contains real stories of real people trying to implement those principles and techniques. Telling the stories from Pittsburgh show what is possible in a small unit, in an institution, or even in a medical specialty. It's also a way of honoring those engaged in the extremely difficult work of change.

---

1. Jeffrey Liker, *The Toyota Way* (New York: McGraw-Hill, 2004).
2. Steven Spear and H. Kent Bowen," Decoding the DNA of the Toyota Production System," *Harvard Business Review* (September 1999).
3. Taiichi Ohno, *Toyota Production System: Beyond Large-Scale Production*, (New York: Productivity, 1988).
4. Cindy Jimmerson, *reVIEW: Realizing Exceptional Value in Everyday Work*, © 2004.

INTRODUCTION

By 2000, when the Institute of Medicine (IOM) released its seminal report, *To Err is Human*,[1] leaders in Pittsburgh had been sitting together for two years, trying to unlock the door to healthcare improvement and cost reduction in Southwestern Pennsylvania.

Nationally, that IOM report kicked off a round of unprecedented soul searching about safety in the healthcare industry. The report shocked the country with the news that as many as 98,000 Americans die from medical mistakes in hospitals each year. Medical error alone, it said, represented the third leading cause of death in the nation.

But the news was about to get worse.

A Centers for Disease Control (CDC) study in 2000 estimated that 2.1 million healthcare-acquired infections occur annually in the United States, causing or contributing to another 88,000 deaths.[2] (These deaths are over and above the 98,000 referred to in the IOM report, which did not define healthcare-acquired infections as "medical errors.")

Meanwhile, fewer and fewer Americans are covered by health insurance. Yet one 2003 study showed that even insured Americans receive the recommended healthcare services for the treatment of their conditions only about half the time.[3]

That this level of care should consume 15 percent of the country's gross domestic product[4] defied comprehension by, among others, the Pittsburgh business community.

---

1. Kohn L., Corrigan J., Donaldson M., (eds), *To Err is Human: Building a Safer Health System.* Committee on Quality Health Care in America, Institute of Medicine, National Academy Press, Washington, D.C., 2000.
2. R. W. Haley et al., CMS 17.29 "The nationwide nosocomial infection rate: a new need for vital statistics," *Am J Epidemiol* 121:159–67, (1985).
3. Elizabeth McGlynn, "The Quality of Health Care Delivered to Adults in the United States," *N Engl J Med* 348:2635–2645, (June 26, 2003).
4. CMS report, cited in *Health Affairs* 23:1, 147–159, Project HOPE, DOI: 10.1377/hlthaff.23.1.147.

PITTSBURGH'S LEADERS ASK THE QUESTIONS

In 1997, three years before the release of the IOM report, a group of business leaders and a local philanthropic organization in Pittsburgh sat down together to discuss ways of "bringing new jobs, capital investment, and a better quality of life to the 10-county region of Southwestern Pennsylvania."[5] This coalition of respected civic leaders, the Allegheny Conference on Community Development, began to look at the business of healthcare—the region's largest economic sector, employing one in eight workers and responsible for more than $7.2 billion in business. The pressure on the healthcare sector had begun showing up as operating losses, bankruptcies, consolidations, and a high rate of employee turnover. From the discussions at the Allegheny Conference emerged the Pittsburgh Regional Health Initiative (PRHI), a nonprofit community consortium designed to respond to these challenges.

PRHI was led by Karen Wolk Feinstein, PhD, president of the Jewish Healthcare Foundation, who recruited former Alcoa Chairman and U.S. Treasury Secretary Paul O'Neill to help lead the consortium. The PRHI convened an array of the region's healthcare stakeholders and posed the question: *Could Southwestern Pennsylvania, working together as a region, create a better healthcare system?*

FOUNDATIONS OF PRHI

The group drafted an ambitious agenda, agreeing that two things needed to be at the core of every medical encounter: patient safety and the provision of the best known care. In other words, from its inception, PRHI based its work on the premise that improving the quality of care would first and foremost save lives, but also revolutionize the business and fiscal health of healthcare. From the beginning, quality was the business case.

That idea—that quality was an important business proposition—had been around in business circles for decades in various guises: Total Quality Management, Continuous Quality Improvement, Six Sigma, and the

5. www.alleghenyconference.org.

Toyota Production System (or Lean). But the underlying premise, that quality was less expensive, was a hard sell in the healthcare community at PRHI's inception a decade ago. Although subsequent work would confirm that hypothesis,[6] at the time, it was presumed by most in the healthcare industry that as healthcare quality increased, so would cost. In considering healthcare cost, quality, and access, it was believed the best that could be attained would be "two out of three."[7]

Still Pittsburgh's leaders persisted. They set ambitious goals for healthcare in Southwestern Pennsylvania, and expressed them in unusually bold terms:

1. Patient safety goals:
   - Zero medication errors.
   - Zero healthcare-acquired (nosocomial) infections.
2. "Perfect" clinical outcomes in the certain areas. (To see how close they came to "perfect," and measure improvement, the group planned to measure complications, like infections, and readmissions—before and after PRHI-led regional working groups tackled the problems.) In the beginning, the clinical areas included coronary artery bypass graft (CABG) surgery; orthopedics (hip and knee replacement); obstetrics (maternal and child outcome); and chronic conditions, starting with depression and diabetes.[8]
3. Adaptation of the Toyota Production System (sometimes called lean thinking) for improving healthcare processes, which became known as Perfecting Patient Care. PRHI would develop a curriculum for teaching these industry-based principles and use examples from the healthcare setting to teach them. This Perfecting

---

6. E. Fisher, MD, MPH, "Medical Care: is more always better?" *N Engl J Med* 349;17:1665–1667 (2004). See also http://www.dartmouthatlas.org/atlases/Vermont_Summit.pdf.
7. Health Law Lecture, Prof. Charity Scott, Georgia State School of Law, 2003.
8. Of the clinical initiatives, the cardiac and chronic care initiatives remain. Orthopedics disbanded for lack of interest. The OB working group exhibited enough vitality to sustain itself, no longer requiring PRHI as a neutral convener.

Patient Care University, a four-day intensive course, would become a community resource, and the curriculum would be available to anyone wishing to pursue it. Cost for the course would be kept low to encourage participation. Furthermore, PRHI would hire coaches trained in the methodology and make them available to selected units throughout the region where the desire for change had been demonstrated.

ZERO

Of all the hopeful—some said naïve—ideas to come out of PRHI in its youth, none provoked more controversy and outright ire than the "zero goal." Many found the notion insulting, believing that what was being demanded of healthcare practitioners—zero errors, or perfection—was humanly unattainable. In the area of healthcare-acquired infections, practitioners at that time believed them to be akin to an "act of God," an inevitable but unfortunate consequence of complicated care.

Over time, the conversation began to shift. The goal of "zero" began to be viewed more from the patient's perspective. To the patient, how many errors are okay? Who would volunteer to be harmed or have harm inflicted on one of their family members in a lottery of harm? And yet, if the only acceptable number of errors is, indeed, zero, how can fallible human beings working within fallible systems begin to approach that goal?

The question evolved from the accusatory, "Why aren't you perfect?" or "Why don't you?" to the more inquiring, "Why can't we?" Instead of blaming individuals who are hard wired to make all-too-human mistakes, why couldn't the underlying system be redesigned to respond to each worker, making it less and less possible for mistakes to occur? These questions formed the basis for adapting the Toyota-based methodology to healthcare. The resulting model set about to improve care at the bedside, one encounter at a time.

A PATIENT IS NOT A CAR

Another provocative idea to emerge from PRHI in its early days was the idea that Perfecting Patient Care, based on Toyota's improvement model, could be applied to healthcare.[9] After all, a patient is not a car, and the infinite variations of the human body, clinicians believed, would not respond to standard practice. The image of patients rolling down an assembly line turned people off.

One of the advantages of the PRHI coalition was the ability of non-healthcare CEOs, from banks and small businesses to industrial giants like Alcoa, to exchange ideas with hospital CEOs and medical practitioners. These conversations led to a hypothesis they viewed worth testing: *perhaps the tenets of an industrial model like the Toyota Production System could be adapted to reduce waste and error in healthcare as dramatically as it has done in industry.*

As the world's leading auto manufacturer, Toyota produces cars of extremely high quality, yet has posted profits every year since 1950. The Toyota or lean system of production is practiced on two levels: the philosophical—valuing the contribution of each worker, continually rooting out waste and defects; and practical—rearranging materials and human resources to support improved efficiency. The result is to use as few resources as possible to produce a product of the highest quality, just in time. Under Paul O'Neill, Alcoa had made use of the Toyota model to make its workplace the safest in the world—and saw a corresponding rise in profits.

In industrial settings, reductions in waste always seemed to lead to reductions in error. It happened at Toyota and again at Alcoa. In the final analysis, work is work, whether it's being performed in a factory or in a hospital. Incremental error reduction should translate to greater and greater safety for patients and a safer, more rewarding work atmosphere for workers.

Could a Toyota-style improvement system make healthcare safer? Perhaps the healthcare system itself could be redesigned in a way that would help reduce waste, prevent errors, improve care, and support workers by making it easy for them to do the right thing and harder to do the wrong

---

9. PRHI initially referred to the improvement methodology as the "Toyota Production System," and Toyota Supplier Support Center (TSSC) provided active support during startup. However, the company eventually voiced concern over using its name in such an organized and wide-ranging endeavor. PRHI was also convinced that the application of these methods to healthcare did indeed create a unique method, and so entitled it "Perfecting Patient Care" and applied for Service Mark (SM) designation.

thing. PRHI adapted the Toyota model to healthcare, entitled it Perfecting Patient Care, and now teaches its techniques.

Initially, hospital units tentatively tried some of the ideas in peripheral areas where waste was undeniable, such as in the organization of supply lines. It made sense to get rid of unused inventory and organize what was there, and in that context, the application of "industrial" techniques did not offend.

Eventually, however, pharmacies and laboratories began to look at their processes and see definite parallels with assembly lines, with possibilities for improvement through standardization of processes. And finally, physicians began to see that applying the techniques clinically, such as to reduce central line-associated bloodstream infections,[10] also worked.

The Perfecting Patient Care University curriculum and on-site coaches remain the distinguishing features of PRHI. Other regional and national efforts have promoted data collection and collaboration among "stakeholders" and competitors, but none has developed an actual on-the-ground method to create dramatic improvement and shared it broadly, not for profit. The class has attracted students from across the nation.

Interestingly, the IOM released a report in 2005 called "Building Better Delivery Systems: A New Engineering/Healthcare Partnership."[11] This report, a joint venture of the National Academy of Engineering and the Institute of Medicine, describes the ways in which engineering discipline aligns with healthcare improvement, leaning heavily on the experiences of PRHI's introduction of Perfecting Patient Care, particularly at the Veterans Administration Pittsburgh Healthcare System (VAPHS).

A REGIONAL LEARNING LABORATORY

From the start, PRHI was envisioned as a collaboration of everyone who had a stake in healthcare in Southwestern Pennsylvania. Using the whole

10. A bloodstream infection caused by the presence of a vascular infusion device (central line) that terminated at or close to the heart or in one of the great vessels. These devices are used to deliver medication or nutrition to the sickest patients, most often in a hospital intensive care unit.
11. National Academy of Engineering (NAE) and Institute of Medicine (IOM), *Building a Better Delivery System: A New Engineering/Health Care Partnership*. (Washington, D.C.: IOM, 2005.)

region seemed to offer a manageable geographic area and market within which to demonstrate the power of perfecting care and removing error. Patients migrate among systems and providers and an entire region offered a logical area for tracking outcomes of care. Southwestern Pennsylvania became a learning lab.

It was assumed that key players would work across competitive boundaries to advance safety and quality for all patients—concepts central to all medical care, and ethically beyond debate. The rules were that institutions would acknowledge problems and share solutions openly among themselves, and all ships would rise. While this worked well in some instances, it created tension in others. Roadblocks were sometimes encountered at various levels of management even though collaborations usually sailed smoothly among frontline staff. Sometimes encouragement from the regional coalition helped; sometimes it didn't.

Sharing failures and solutions is not easy for bitter competitors. However, PRHI was successful in establishing convenient local learning networks and performance improvement coalitions. Institutions have learned and borrowed best practices from one another and even exchanged observational visits.

Today it seems less remarkable to have a team from Allegheny General going to observe infection control practices at the VAPHS, or to have nurses from Family Services of Western Pennsylvania going to observe at a Children's Hospital UPMC clinic to see how to schedule first appointments more effectively. PRHI no longer needs to take an active role in promoting cross-institutional visits; more and more, they just occur. The region is becoming a learning laboratory.

THE DILEMMA OF SPREAD

"The one reality of the Toyota Way is that there is always more than one way to achieve the desired result."[12]

Like other organizations striving to improve patient safety, PRHI struggled to find the quickest route to institutional transformation. Traditionally,

---

12. J. Liker and D. Meier, *The Toyota Way Fieldbook: A Practical Guide for Implementing Toyota's 4Ps* (New York: McGraw-Hill 2006).

the Toyota system requires that an entire entity—a whole company or industry, for example—commit to doing work in this new way. The organization and its work culture are made over in the process. Anything less than full commitment to a new way of working risks introducing the tools without the strategy—contrary to the strictest interpretation of the Toyota way.

For PRHI to have any impact, its teachers and coaches had to be invited in by institutions willing to try something new. PRHI leadership began offering classroom training and coaches to work in the trenches beside employees at the point of care, solving problems one by one using the Perfecting Patient Care model. Giving workers a say in how their work is designed, they believed, would be the shortest route to institutional transformation.

Such a transformation begins with an understanding of the Toyota principles that Spear and Bowen call Rules in Use,[13] or as PRHI calls them, the Rules of Work Redesign (see sidebar). These principles specify activities, connections, and pathways of work, and specify how to experiment with improvements. The more these principles were accepted by a broad range of leaders—especially top leaders—the more widely and quickly the ideas spread. PRHI coaches began teaching the principles in a classroom and on the floor, in real-world situations.

Instead of trying to institute sweeping, wall-to-wall institutional transformations up front, these efforts started wherever they could. Improvements may have begun tentatively, with process improvements in one unit, for example. The idea was to pilot the work, show rapid process improvement, and sustain it—thereby demonstrating the value of the ideas in healthcare. Building a better mousetrap would surely attract more interest. Improving a process was often the first step in redesigning a whole system.

In several cases, it worked that way. Some leaders showed willingness to take the principles across the organization. For example, the work against infection that PRHI helped develop at the VAPHS was recently adopted nationwide. In another example of spread, a group of pathologists

---

13. H. Kent Bowen and Steven Spear, "Decoding the DNA of the Toyota Production System." (HBS Working Knowledge for Business Leaders, October 12, 1999.)

The Rules of Work Redesign, derived from Bowen and Spear's "Rules in Use," guide process improvement in Perfecting Patient Care℠.

Rule 1: Activities (work) must be highly specified as to content, sequence, timing, location and expected outcome.

Rule 2: Connections between customers and suppliers must be highly specified, direct, with a clear yes-or-no way to send requests and receive responses.

Rule 3: The pathway for every product and service must be predefined, highly specified, simple and direct—no loops or forks.

Rule 4: Improvements are made using the scientific method, with guidance from a teacher, as close as possible to the work, aiming toward the ideal.

Specify each design . . . Test each use . . . Improve with each problem. Fill in this statement to get started: Ideally, we would like to [. . . .], but this problem is in our way. We will design a temporary improvement, and experiment with it until our work comes as close as possible to the ideal.

decided to apply the principles to revolutionize their specialty, and that work has spread from Pittsburgh to Detroit. Over time, many hospitals, community organizations, and even physicians' offices began to change.

But implementing system improvements, whether through Perfecting Patient Care or other means, is exceptionally difficult. A given plan doesn't always take off. Some who have taken the Perfecting Patient Care University courses, for example, report going back to their institutions, observing problems, and suggesting system changes, only to collide with peer attitudes that reflect an institution ill-equipped to accept change. Even when a better mousetrap was built, it often remained confined to one unit or team.

Only when physicians and top leaders themselves championed the work did lasting improvements result and spread within institutions and the community. Several of the case studies in this book demonstrate what happens when top leaders become committed.

Acting on the realization that leadership engagement was all, in 2006, PRHI and its parent organization, the Jewish Healthcare Foundation, created two programs to accelerate quality improvement across the region:

the Nurse Navigator and Physician Champion programs. Nine nurses and eight physicians received training in the principles of Perfecting Patient Care. Each received a small stipend to compensate for the training time. For one year, each team pursued a quality-improvement project in which they held an abiding interest. Several of these projects are profiled here.

THE REIMBURSEMENT SYSTEM: A PREREQUISITE TO TRANSFORMATIONAL CHANGE

When PRHI began its work, conventional wisdom said that improvements in quality would be too costly. The Pittsburgh experiments have shown that the opposite is true. Higher quality leads to lower cost.

Improvements unequivocally save lives *and money*. One study showed hospitals saving thousands of dollars when central line-associated bloodstream infections were eliminated.[14] But eventually the question devolves to, "Whose money is being saved?" Insurers'? Hospitals'? Physicians'?

Stymieing broad-scale improvement is the current reimbursement system, which many have called toxic. In some cases, increased efficiency actually leads to a punishing decrease in income. In January 2007, the *Wall Street Journal*[15] described a case at Virginia Mason Hospital in Seattle. That hospital found a better way to treat patients with back pain, referring them to physical therapy first, rather than recommending and repeating expensive MRIs and specialist visits. Patients got better quicker, and the insurers saved hundreds of dollars per patient: However, Virginia Mason lost money, in effect, being punished for becoming more efficient. Only one insurer agreed to increase reimbursement in exchange for the improved efficiency.

"Insurers often reimburse high-tech procedures richly, while simpler remedies and visits to doctors, therapists or nurses earn far less and sometimes incur losses," said the article. "Even Medicare has experimented

---

14. R. Shannon et al., "Economics of Central Line-Associated Bloodstream Infections," *American Journal of Medical Quality* 21:6 suppl, 7S–16S (2006).
15. Vanessa Fuhrmans, "A Novel Plan Helps Hospital Wean Itself Off Pricey Tests," *Wall Street Journal*, page 1, January 12, 2007.

recently with performance bonuses, to correct a system that it acknowledges 'rewards volume over quality.'"

It is not enough to acknowledge that efficiency will save money: The reimbursement system must change. Today PRHI is shifting its focus toward a more thorough examination of the medical reimbursement system and possible solutions. It is a daunting task, and will involve regional coalitions from across the country.

CASE STUDIES AS PROFILES IN COURAGE

This book serves as a field guide describing how Perfecting Patient Care strategies have been implemented in various medical settings throughout a community. The stories demonstrate what can happen when a respected, nonprofit, neutral entity joins the business community in offering education and brokering change in the healthcare delivery system, for the benefit of the community at large and each of its citizens.

In the beginning, many hospitals seemed suspicious of this new "industrial" approach advocated by PRHI, and decided to "try" it in one unit, or on one problem. The effort may well have died there. However, Pittsburgh had its bully pulpit in PRHI and its Board. PRHI's parent organization, the Jewish Healthcare Foundation, along with the Veterans Administration, Centers for Disease Control and Prevention, and the Agency for Healthcare Research and Quality, continued to fund these improvement experiments across the region, not only in hospitals, but in community and other nonprofit health organizations.

Underlying the stories in this volume is the perseverance of many leaders in Pittsburgh's healthcare and nonprofit communities who still are working to transform healthcare delivery in Southwestern Pennsylvania through the method known as Perfecting Patient Care. PRHI CEO Karen Wolk Feinstein, PhD, summarizes it this way: "It has been extremely difficult for the clinicians and quality champions featured in this book to persevere in the present culture. All around them are peers, management, and institutions facing concerns about the unintended consequences of QI . . . fear of litigation from transparency, loss of patients, institutional recrimination, anger of peers, loss of income, public media exposure, and trustee loss of confidence. They were swimming upstream, risking careers and leadership positions. However, in spite of all this, they found that change in the form of Perfecting Patient Care, for them and their peers, was not extra work, but a liberating removal of wasted efforts from inefficiencies and errors."

These stories illustrate that careful, systematic, incremental improvements, such as creating reliable supply lines, can indeed fuel more complex improvements, such as eliminating infections. They demonstrate that one "simple" improvement, like reducing falls or making wheelchairs widely available, ultimately cannot be corralled in a single unit, but necessarily involves the whole organization. They show that certain improvements, like a standardized form to make shift change more efficient, will spread like wildfire once other units discover them. Over time, transformation of an entire organization may start with a single effort in a single unit, if the leadership supports the effort, and these improvements will be sustained.

Perhaps most important, these stories demonstrate that every staff member is the expert in what they do, and that it takes everyone, backed by top leaders, to make improvements that stick. The improvements require mutual respect and a certain degree of autonomy—traits of a healthy workplace[16] that serve patients and employees well.

---

16. H. K. Spence and J. Finegan, "Empowering Nurses for Work Engagement and Health in Hospital Settings," *JONA: The Journal of Nursing Administration*. Front material, May 10, 2007.

CHAPTER 1

Why it Matters

When you hear the numbers—100,000 American lives lost each year due to medical mishaps and another 90,000 to hospital-acquired infection—it's easy to feel hopeless. It's easy to write off any hope for change, to assign blame. It is easy to depersonalize the story, blurring the edges with statistics instead of looking at the stories: living, breathing people and their families.

Even when healthcare professionals seek care for themselves or their families, they find the current system nonnavigable. This chapter details an exceedingly personal story intended to describe, in excruciating detail, why healthcare improvement matters: *because every medical statistic has a face.*

MEET THE LARES

For Steve and Diane Lares, it was indeed a wonderful life. In 1998, at the age of 37, Steve had completed his doctorate and, after serving as a high-school principal, had worked his way up to assistant superintendent. With his stellar professional credentials, he was applying to various institutions for superintendent positions.

After receiving her degree in medical science and an MBA, Diane had made a career transition from physician assistant to healthcare consultant with the Pennsylvania Medical Society. The Lares family lived in a small Southwestern Pennsylvania town with their two daughters, 13-year-old Karen and 9-year-old Kristen.

"We had the brick house, two kids, two-car garage, church involvement, a camper—a rich and busy life," said Diane.

But life came unraveled one day in 1998, when Diane noticed that the right side of Steve's face was drooping strangely. The diagnosis could not have been more devastating: *glioblastoma multiforme*, a particularly aggressive brain cancer. With this kind of cancer, it's not so much a question of a five-year survival rate: Few people survive even three years.

Steve and Diane prepared for the fight of their lives. Surely Diane's knowledge of medicine and the healthcare system could help ensure that Steve received the best of care. However, reality soon intruded.

"All of a sudden, our lives turned upside down. The healthcare system just made us more perplexed and frustrated," she said. "Even with my knowledge and 'connections,' I could not make the healthcare system work for my family."

Six and a half months

In the ensuing six and a half months, between his diagnosis and his death, Steve endured seven surgeries. He was a patient in more than one hospital. Together, Steve and Diane endured the frustrations of a broken healthcare system, as his care degenerated into a cascade of errors that Diane was powerless to anticipate or fix.

This story could have happened anywhere. It wasn't a matter of one "bad hospital" or one "bad doctor," but rather an entire system in chaos, having lost its focus on the basics of care, respect, and dignity for the patient.

First, to assess the tumor and plan for radiation treatment, Steve needed an MRI, but the utilization review company in New Jersey had to approve it. Each day of delay in the planning meant a week's delay in radiation treatment. With the disease's relentless timeline, each day was unbearably precious. Finally, they were reduced to begging. To a voice on the other end of the line, an emotional Steve pleaded, "You don't realize, I have two small daughters I need to live for."

At last the company relented.

Overwhelmed nurses

Diane often saw nurses rushing in to do their job, taking Steve's blood pressure and scurrying off. They lacked time to provide the level of care that they as professionals, and Steve as a patient, deserved. Occasionally the nurses, knowing of Diane's medical background, would ask her to tell hospital administrators that they needed more staff.

Whenever Steve was hospitalized, Diane often stayed at his bedside. She was puzzled when, one night, the nurses began to bathe Steve in the middle of the night. Only later did it occur to Diane that this had been an intentional tactic to dissuade her from staying all night. It was galling to realize that, in the view of some nurses, families were simply in the way.

Diane arrived at the hospital one day to find Steve's face bruised, his nose scratched. He had fallen. After being brought back from physical therapy, he had been placed in his room in a wheelchair, out of reach of a call bell. Before the nurse could make it back to check on him, he needed to use the bathroom and did not realize that he could not make it by himself. The nurse felt almost as bad as Steve looked.

Steve joked, "Michelle does not think it is funny when her patients fall. She doesn't have a sense of humor about my adventure at all."

Diagnosis and prognosis

The healthcare team repeatedly assured Diane and Steve that the tumor was shrinking. With her medical knowledge, though, Diane just couldn't figure out why the healthcare team was doing things the way they were. The treatment plan didn't make sense until a young intern surreptitiously admitted why: Steve's tumor had actually enlarged. The intern did not have permission to tell either patient or family. It was supposed to be a secret—*from them!*

Later, during six weeks of radiation therapy, the family was delighted when the surgeon told them that this time, the radiation was killing the tumor. Yet Steve's right-sided weakness grew progressively worse. Finally, the surgeon admitted that he had not actually measured the tumor each visit, but had just "eyeballed" it. In truth, the tumor was growing—dramatically. To the devastated couple he offered only a shrug.

Diane and Steve craved human connections, respect, and dignity, but instead felt like cogs in some machine. After one surgery, Diane noticed that the surgeon had scrawled the name, "Charlton Heston" across the bandage around Steve's head. When Diane asked why, the assistants chuckled and explained that it was a joke.

As if to ameliorate the indignity, one assistant added, "He writes Marilyn Monroe on the women's head bandages."

Today, Diane is still haunted that she allowed her husband to lie there, the object of a joke, until his next dressing change. But she knew that being the "angry family member" only risks further alienating the staff.

"It still bothers me that I did not express outrage," says Diane. "But you feel so vulnerable."

To drive home the point that Steve was still a person, and therefore worth saving, Diane brought snapshots taken before his illness to the doctor's visits. Whenever the girls came to the hospital, Diane made sure they were scrubbed to effulgence, dressed in their Sunday clothes. They learned to "dress up, so Daddy can get better care."

"I felt obligated for us to be the nice, undemanding family," she said.

Hospital-acquired infection

Following one of his seven surgeries, Steve contracted a postoperative, hospital-acquired infection of the bone flap. This meant six weeks of a powerful intravenous (IV) antibiotic administered every 12 hours, at home, many times dispensed by Karen, their 13-year-old daughter.

Home-health nurses fretted when the IV supplies where not "organized the way they should be." The criticism stung.

"We felt as if they were invading our home when they came," said Diane. "They noticed the dust bunnies, but did not appear to see us as a family in crisis, dealing with a tragedy."

In one particularly harrowing episode, Diane rushed Steve to the hospital with a severe headache and vomiting due to the swelling in his head. She parked by the entrance of a large city hospital and ran in for help as Steve lay curled in pain on the front seat of the car.

There he remained for the half hour it took to find a wheelchair.

Later, Diane sat beside Steve for hours in the emergency department, now in a fetal position, as his head pain intensified. A staff member finally acknowledged why they were refusing, after all that time, to give him pain medication: "We don't have an order."

Diane argued with the physician covering the floor that Memorial Day weekend. Steve was having brain-stem herniation, an incredibly painful displacement of brain tissue and fluids outside of their normal locations in the head. It is a serious, but common, secondary effect of a brain tumor. That weekend, they were treating the pain, but not the swelling, which was its cause. Diane asked the on-call cancer specialist why he was not working to reduce the swelling. He replied that his specialty was breast cancer, not brain cancer. He was just covering the cancer service for the weekend.

Planning for the unthinkable

Was Steve actively dying? Diane and Steve asked their physician for a realistic prognosis. With a family to protect, they found themselves facing the painful dichotomy of clinging to life while planning for death. They scheduled and rescheduled a meeting, but the physician repeatedly cancelled. Finally, a member of the staff told Diane that this doctor didn't like to talk about death. It meant failure and defeat—*for him.*

In the absence of a frank discussion of death, Steve reverted to his underlying positive attitude: He focused on living. Soon, well-intentioned caregivers began to whisper to Diane that Steve must be in denial, because he was not ready for hospice talk.

In truth, Diane and Steve had accepted that he would die of brain cancer, and probably soon. But the emotional journey from diagnosis to impending death was passing with blinding speed, and it encompassed periods of shock, disbelief, and paralysis. Perhaps because of Diane's medical background, nobody on the care team thought to discuss sincerely with her the specifics of what could happen, and what choices, exactly, she might need to make for Steve. Everyone figured she, of all people, would know exactly what to do. But when "the patient" is a beloved family member, judgment can be colored by the sheer desire for that life to continue in any form, at any cost.

A bolt from the blue

On a cold Saturday in January 1999, Diane arrived at the hospital to visit. The plan was to bring Steve home after a six-week hospitalization. The tumor was under control and he was, at the moment, stable. She had spent all morning cleaning the house and had stopped by the bakery for treats.

"The moment I arrived at the hospital, I knew that something wasn't right," said Diane. "I kept asking everyone what was going on and was told they weren't sure but they'd called the physician, and he had given orders. Steve was short of breath. Things were getting worse."

That evening the resident on call urged Diane to have a breathing tube installed, so that the act of breathing wouldn't exhaust Steve. Her only thought was, "Please don't let him suffocate."

Walking to the nurses' station for a break, she overheard the nurse say, "I don't know, Doctor, I don't know why she made that decision." Diane inquired what was wrong? The nurse replied, "Steve's doctor doesn't think he should have been intubated."

When the physician arrived—the same one who had refused to discuss end-of-life issues with the couple—he was clearly agitated, huffing angrily, "I guess we will have to transfer him to the ICU now!"

During the transfer, Diane overheard the physician say, "He probably has a pulmonary embolus, but I'm not sure why. He was on heparin." Diane knew this meant a serious blood clot had formed in Steve's lung, in spite of the fact that he had been prescribed a strong blood-thinning medicine.

Then a nurse said, "No, you never reordered the heparin. He has been off it for the past couple of days, because we thought you wanted it stopped." The clot had formed because the blood-thinner in Steve's system was below therapeutic levels.

All alone in the hallway outside of the ICU waiting room, Diane calmly waited for word. She knew that a pulmonary embolus, while serious, was treatable. The surgeon approached, asking whether she would want the team to run a "code" to restart Steve's heart if it should stop. And just like that, the crucial moment was upon her. After all the planning, it struck like a bolt from the blue.

Diane said, "Of course you should code him! The tumor is under control. We are planning to go home. We were talking just a few hours ago."

The doctor walked off, gesticulating in disgust. Diane called after him, "Is that the wrong decision?"

Later, Diane would learn that Steve's heart had already stopped before the surgeon asked the question.

"He asked me later how long I wanted them to run the code," said Diane. "I told them to use the typical standard, 'Until you know it is hopeless.' He told me I was being barbaric. I was in total disbelief at what was happening."

When Diane's parents arrived, the physician started to plead his case with them, despite Diane's pleas to leave them out of it. Finally, after some private moments of family discussion, they agreed that the code could stop.

Soon the girls arrived, expecting to accompany their father home. They had just stepped off the hospital elevator when Diane took them aside. Their screams echoed through the halls.

On the way out of the hospital, Diane stopped back at the unit to gather Steve's belongings and told the nurse that she was upset with how the situation had been handled. The nurse seemed to feel awkward.

"One moment of awkwardness," said Diane, "and that was the end of Steve's story for them."

The aftermath

It was not the end of the story for Diane. It took nearly a year before she could resolve the avalanche of bills, most of which were wrong. Struggling through grief, and learning to get by on a single paycheck, Diane endured sleepless nights making draconian financial contingency plans as more bills filled her mailbox. Among the erroneous claims:

- A bill from the surgeon for $10,000 with a message, highlighted in yellow, demanding, "Please pay immediately."
- An explanation of benefits that rejected an entire hospitalization (after his death) that said, "Employee's responsibility: $155,000."
- Bills for Steve's radiation therapy, totaling tens of thousands, stating that it had not been administered by an approved participating provider.

Perhaps the most painful aspect of Steve's death for Diane was the knowledge that he hadn't died of the brain tumor, but from mismanagement of his anticoagulation medication—a classic medication error.

"What seemed the most unbelievable, even to me, a healthcare professional, was how big a struggle it was to get the right care. Of course, many wonderful people cared for Steve. There is no one to blame," she says. "It is because of fragmentation and complexity that most of these things happened. Members of the healthcare community seem to throw their hands up and say that it will be impossible to fix it. But I know we can design a better healthcare system. We must prevent infections, errors, and get back to the real purpose of healthcare. It is because of my husband, and countless other family members who die needlessly or too soon, that we need to redesign the system. All people who need healthcare deserve a system designed around their needs—regardless of who they are."

Bitter or better?

Refusing to blame or be consumed by anger, Diane heeded the words of her pastoral counselor, who told her, "You can become bitter. Or you can become better."

Although she was told she could (or even should) file a lawsuit, Diane did not. Doing so would only have prolonged her anger, and her daughters needed her strength, not her rage. She needed time and understanding to heal, not money. Besides, she reasoned, if lawsuits really taught the desired lessons, if they really improved healthcare, then healthcare would surely be perfect by now. Her research told her that lawsuits only serve to drive problems deeper underground instead of exposing them to the light of day where they can be solved. All of her reading told her that a "blame-free culture," which is so foreign to healthcare, is essential for improvement. She refused to fuel a culture of blame.

So Diane decided to live her life with a new mission: making healthcare safer. Two years after Steve's death, Diane began working with the Pittsburgh Regional Health Initiative (PRHI) as the curriculum expert for the Perfecting Patient Care^{SM} University. She pioneered the first university curriculum adapting the basics of the Toyota Production System specifically for healthcare workers, and taught it for three years. She changed minds. She changed lives. She began to heal. She remarried. The girls are thriving.

Today, Diane is a vice president of organizational excellence with a local hospital system—one of the places where Steve's illness took him. She is still striving to help the system work better than ever.

"At first it was difficult to walk into a hospital where Steve had been," said Diane. "The memories were still painful. But this is where I have an opportunity to make a difference by touching lives—with Steve's story and because of many others' stories of people who need true healthcare."

THE POWER OF THE STORY

Storytelling is one of the most powerful ways human beings can communicate. While the story of the Lares family evokes strong emotions—sadness for the family, sympathy for overworked caregivers, outrage at a broken system—it also serves to set the stage for the stories that follow in the next chapters.

In the following stories, you will see healthcare heroes working to remedy many of the very things that the Lares family endured: hospital-acquired infections, falls, medication errors, nonstandard care, waiting for test results, waiting for appointments, waiting for a wheelchair. Healthcare workers enter their professions to help and to heal. The journey to quality is the journey toward safety for patients, and the promise of fulfillment for workers.

CHAPTER 2

Tackling Hospital-Acquired Infections

CASE STUDIES

- **Section 1. Regional project reduces infections.** When 30 Pittsburgh-area hospitals pooled their knowledge and determination, central line-associated bloodstream infections (CLABs) declined by 63 percent over four years.
- **Section 2. Eliminating central line infections within 90 days.** In an effort led by one physician, Perfecting Patient Care techniques all but eliminate central line infections in two intensive care units within 90 days.
- **Section 3. Sustaining the gain against central line infection.** When one inspiring leader leaves the organization after a major gain, how can it be sustained? (Quick answer: find another physician leader.)
- **Section 4. Reducing antibiotic-resistant infections.** A sustained, wide-ranging Perfecting Patient Care program at the VA Pittsburgh Healthcare System reduced a strain of antibiotic-resistant infection (methicillin-resistant *Staphylococcus aureus* or MRSA) by more than 85 percent.
- **Section 5. Redesigning a system: the wheelchairs.** It's an emotional issue among staff. Will there be a wheelchair when my patient needs one? Will it be the right configuration? Will it be clean? Wheelchair availability and cleanliness are system issues, requiring the application of Perfecting Patient Care throughout the entire VA Pittsburgh Healthcare System.

SHEDDING LIGHT ON STATISTICS

Hospitals are places of miraculous healing and heroic care. However, as with any human-led endeavor, there are problems. According to the Centers for Disease Control and Prevention (CDC), about one in ten hospitalized patients acquires an infection after being admitted to the hospital.[1] Steve Lares was but one of over 2 million people who contracted a hospital-acquired infection in the course of his care in 1997. The CDC estimates that 90,000 people die from infections, and that they add billions of dollars in healthcare costs. These infections are associated with increased mortality, length of stay, hospital costs, and antibiotic resistance.

Yet even today, few American hospitals can cite their rates of MRSA infection, just to name one kind of pervasive, generally hospital-acquired infection.

To date, 43 states either have enacted or are considering legislation to require hospitals to report their infection rates publicly. Pennsylvania has already begun to do so. These factors, along with expanding media coverage, are converging to make hospital-acquired infections a mainstream *cause célèbre*, not only among clinical patient safety advocates, but also among consumer groups and the general public. Calls for full public disclosure of infection rates, and for the eradication of infections in the nation's hospitals have appeared in lay literature as diverse as *Consumer Reports* and *Slate Magazine*.

It wasn't always so.

In 2001, when the Pittsburgh Regional Health Initiative (PRHI) first tackled the two most prevalent hospital-acquired infections, one associated with central line catheters, the other with antibiotic-resistant bacteria, the medical establishment was loath to label infections "medical errors." Nevertheless, PRHI's regional partners decided to ignore the labels, join hands, and bring down the rates of these infections, through systematic information sharing, and by whatever process means they chose. The case studies in this chapter describe those results.

---

1. R. P. Plowman, N. Graves, and J. A. Roberts. Hospital acquired infection. (London: Office of Health Economics, 1997).

• SECTION 1 •

REGIONAL PROJECT REDUCES INFECTIONS

Sometimes just bringing a problem to light and discussing it will start improvements rolling. Starting in 2001, the Pittsburgh Regional Health Initiative[2] (PRHI) convened infection-control practitioners and infectious-disease physicians from across the region and across competing healthcare systems in meetings. These professionals shared ideas as a collective working group about the best practices for preventing the spread of infection.

Specifically, the group was working to eliminate central line-associated bloodstream infections in the region's intensive care units. Central lines are tiny catheters placed in major vessels that deliver life-saving medication or nutrition directly into the bloodstreams of critically ill patients—and conversely, when handled improperly, efficiently deliver the microorganisms that cause systemic bloodstream infections. Pittsburgh's community-wide effort was also supported by the Centers for Disease Control and Prevention (CDC), which published guidelines in the prevention of central line infections in 2002.[3]

How serious are these hospital-acquired bloodstream infections? Because central lines are generally inserted in the sickest patients, those infections are among the deadliest. The Centers for Disease Control and Prevention (CDC) estimates that 250,000 such infections occur in the nation's hospitals each year, with an estimated mortality of 12 percent to 25 percent for each one.[4] Two intensive care units at Allegheny General Hospital, performing a retrospective chart review, put the estimated

---

2. For this infection reduction program, PRHI worked under the auspices of the Centers for Disease Control and Prevention (CDC), with a grant from the Agency for Healthcare Research and Quality (AHRQ).
3. http://www.cdc.gov/ncidod/dhqp/gl_intravascular.html.
4. CDC. Guidelines for the prevention of intravascular catheter-related infections. *MMWR* 5 (No. RR-10): 1–26 (2002).

mortality for central line infections closer to 50 percent.[5] Each infection is estimated to cost between $3,700 and $29,000.[6]

WORRY ABOUT "ZERO" AND BLAME

Many participants feared that adopting a goal of "zero infections"—whether it was achievable or not—would raise expectations to the point that they would be personally blamed for every infection that occurred. Nevertheless, the practitioners kept sharing their best practices, and reporting their infection data to the neutral CDC every quarter on one type of healthcare-acquired infection: the central line-associated bloodstream infection.

Some infection control experts in the consortium expressed interest in learning about the new Perfecting Patient Care techniques, by taking PRHI-sponsored classes, and asking for on-site help. It was a novel regional approach, adapting industrial improvement practices to healthcare. Perfecting Patient Care prevents infections by improving the design and flow of work and eliminating potential errors. Engaging frontline caregivers to examine mishaps immediately and implement preventive measures are the hallmark of this method. Other elements included staff training about infection control measures, prevention checklists, hospital unit feedback on infection rates, and adherence to appropriate preventive practices.

ENCOURAGING RESULTS OVER TIME

Whether through new, efficient measures or other means, hospitals began to post encouraging results. Quarter after quarter, up to 28 of 39 participating hospitals turned in their infection data (Figure 2-1, and Table 2-1). And quarter after quarter the numbers showed an overall regional decline. Between the third quarter of 2001 and the fourth quarter of 2004, the

---

5. R. Shannon, D. Frndak, and N. Grunden, "Using Real-Time Problem Solving to Eliminate Central Line Infections," *Joint Commission Journal on Quality and Patient Safety* 32:9, (Sept. 2006).
6. S. Verghese et al., "Central venous catheter related infections," *Journal of Communicable Diseases* 31:1–4, (Mar. 1999).

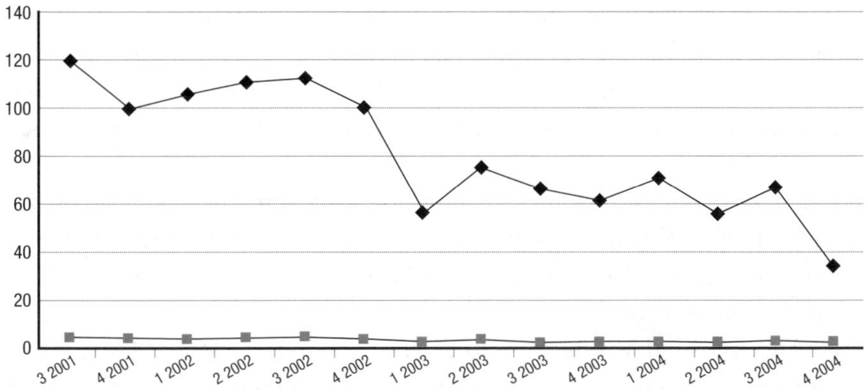

Figure 2-1. The decline wasn't a straight line every quarter, but the general direction was down. In three years, the region posted a 63 percent decline in the central line infection rate. The data were fed to the CDC, then to a local data coordinating center. In this way, hospitals could participate but have their data remain blinded.

Table 2-1. Number of Hospitals Reporting and Number of Central Line Infections in ICUs Quarterly

Quarter/ Year	# CLABs	# of Hospitals Submitting	Rate per 1,000 Line Days
Q3/2001	123	28	4.3
Q4/2001	100	28	3.6
Q1/2002	106	28	3.5
Q2/2002	114	28	4.1
Q3/2002	116	29	3.8
Q4/2002	98	28	3.7
Q1/2003	68	28	2.5
Q2/2003	91	28	3.6
Q3/2003	65	23	2.5
Q4/2003	61	26	2.3
Q1/2004	69	28	2.4
Q2/2004	58	29	1.9
Q3/2004	65	27	2.4
Q4/2004	36	23	1.6

region's hospitals posted a 63 percent decline in the number of central line infections.[7] The number of infections reported by participating hospitals dropped from 123 infections per quarter to 36—a reduction in rate from 4.3 to 1.6 infections per 1,000 patient days at risk because of the presence of a catheter.

"These data demonstrate what can be achieved when bold goals are set, infections are examined one-by-one for causes, and lessons are shared between caregivers without the fear of blame," said Peter Perreiah, then-managing director of PRHI.

CDC Medical Epidemiologist, John Jernigan, MD, added, "The healthcare stakeholders in Southwestern Pennsylvania have challenged the traditional, by setting a goal of eliminating healthcare-associated infections throughout the region. By questioning the limits of what is achievable, healthcare facilities in Pittsburgh have been able to significantly improve patient safety in the entire region."

Achieving a 63 percent decline over many hospitals took four years. Because the study ended in 2004, further data have not been collected, so it is not known whether the regional decline has continued or been sustained. However, several individual hospital units across the region continue to post zero or very few central line infections. The following example is a case in point, where a decline of over 95 percent in central line infections took place within 90 days.

---

7. C. Sirio et al., "Reduction in Central Line–Associated Bloodstream Infections Among Patients in Intensive Care Units—Pennsylvania, April 2001–March 2005," *JAMA*. Vol. 295 No. 3 (January 18, 2006).

"In 2001, CDC was invited by the Pittsburgh Regional Healthcare Initiative (PRHI) to provide technical assistance for a hospital-based intervention to prevent central line–associated bloodstream infections (CLABs) among intensive care unit (ICU) patients in southwestern Pennsylvania. During a 4-year period, BSI rates among ICU patients declined 63 percent, from 4.31 to 1.36 per 1,000 central line days. The results suggest that a coordinated, multiinstitutional infection-control initiative might be an effective approach to reducing healthcare-associated infections."

• SECTION 2 •

ELIMINATING CENTRAL LINE INFECTIONS WITHIN 90 DAYS

Richard Shannon, MD, was Medical Department Chairman at Allegheny General Hospital in 2004, when he became interested in applying Toyota-based Perfecting Patient Care methodology to an actual clinical process. He rejected the common notion that some hospital-acquired infections were an inevitable part of care in a complex medical organization. He had seen impressive improvements at the VA Pittsburgh, as PRHI led a program to standardize processes and supplies on units and watched as the rate of antibiotic-resistant infections declined (Section 3, this chapter).

Shannon decided to take the course offered by PRHI to learn how to apply Perfecting Patient Care directly to the problem of central line-associated bloodstream infections. Hospitals across the entire region were pursuing this problem together: He wanted to test whether or not using these principles could accelerate improvements.

Shannon had become frustrated with the pace of change in medicine. The Centers for Disease Control (CDC) guidelines for central line placement had come out in 2002,[8] yet adoption had been painfully slow. Data on central line infections were retrospective—often six months old or more—and reported in an obscure statistical way. Instead of detailing specifically how many infections occurred or in how many patients, the data are reported in "line days of care," or the total number of days a central line is in place for each patient. Reporting the data that way obscures and depersonalizes the problem.

"Exactly how many *people* is 5.1 infections per 1,000 line days?" Shannon asked.

Retrospective data also made it impossible to root out variation in the process that led to the infection in the first place.

Shannon believed that the scientific method could be applied quickly and continuously if real-time data were disseminated, and acted upon,

8. N. O'Grady et al., "Guidelines for the prevention of intravascular catheter-related infections," *MMWR* Recomm Rep 51(RR-10):1–29 (Aug. 9, 2002).

each time a lab test disclosed an infection. Shannon set an audacious goal: eliminating central line-associated bloodstream infections on the two intensive care units he supervised, (the Medical ICU or MICU, and Coronary Care Unit or CCU) within 90 days.

1. *Establish the current condition.* To find the true dimension of the current problem, Shannon's team conducted a chart review of more than 1,700 MICU and CCU patients who had received central lines during the prior year (2002–2003), when conventional approaches were used. They decided to decode the generic way of reporting, which put the number of infections at 5.1 per 1,000 line days—certainly not higher than at any other time, and not high enough to raise eyebrows.

   When the team members, representing a cross-section of everyone who worked on the floor, analyzed the "line days of care," they discovered that 37 people had contracted central line infections in the prior year, some contracting more than one. Nineteen of those patients died (51 percent). Although some argued that the patients were chronically ill and probably would have died anyway, Shannon's team established that the group with central line infections had nearly double the chance of dying compared to other ICU patients.

   The knowledge that half of the infected patients would die galvanized the nursing staff in a way that no other statistic could have. Nurse leadership from that time forward inspired Shannon to call them the "guardian angels of the central lines."

   From the beginning, Shannon believed it was important to establish zero infections as the goal. The group's research had revealed, for example, that the reported infection rate of 5.1 per 1,000 line days did not include infections of the lines inserted in the femoral, or groin, area, but only those placed in the neck and shoulder (jugular or subclavian) areas. At that time, the CDC did not define femoral line infections as central line infections. If they had, the rate of reported infections in the MICU and CCU during the prior year would have doubled, to 10.5 infections per 1,000 line days. Shannon established early on that the MICU and CCU would track femoral line infections.

"Bacteria don't care which agency defines them, or what kind of line they ride in to the patient," said Shannon. "It is easier to broaden the definition to include *all* infections, and go after them one by one as they occur."

Shannon established one definition: A "central line infection" would be an infection of any central line in the MICU and CCU, including femoral lines. And the goal would be zero.

2. *Observe the actual work in detail, over time.* Shannon and clinically trained staff members from PRHI conducted more than 40 hours of observation. They noted procedures followed during line placements, line maintenance (such as dressing changes), and subtle factors such as communication used during these activities. They noted, among other things, that femoral lines took far longer to dress than subclavian lines.

   But mainly, the observations revealed variations in practice among nurses and doctors that became the basis for standardization.
3. *Use real-time data and act on it immediately with every symptomatic patient.* The retrospective chart review was useful in establishing the current condition. After that, however, the team reverted to real-time data from the laboratory. If an infection was revealed, staff members sped to the bedside of the patient within about six hours to determine why—to find, in the parlance of process improvement, the "root cause." Ordinarily, they discovered one or more steps in the new protocol had been breached, and they set about to find out why. (One of the techniques associated with Perfecting Patient Care is to ask "Why?" five times to discover the root cause of a problem. Doing so increases the likelihood that the team will work to fix the right problem, not an offshoot or subproblem.) Answers to those questions led to collaborative changes in procedures and further staff education.

   Significantly, Shannon made it clear that nurses would have the right and responsibility to stop a procedure if a physician were not following proper procedures. The ability of anyone in the hierarchy to call out defects and stop a procedure is a key safety system used in aviation, analogous to the industrial notion of stopping the assembly line rather than producing a defective

The "Whys" in Action

Often, when a problem arises, say, a nurse cannot find the right syringe in the drawer, the temptation is to fix that problem at that moment, without regard for how it happened. Perhaps that solves the problem for the next one or two rounds, but it will inevitably recur unless the root problem is solved. It's analogous to treating a symptom while the disease rages.

In this case, the Toyota-based Perfecting Patient Care approach raised the awareness, which led to the discovery of the root cause: Asking the question, "Why?" up to five times, boring ever deeper into the problem, uncovers the root cause. When that problem is solved (usually it's a more complex problem than the symptom that presents itself), the entire issue will go away. Because the solution involves changing the way the work is done, backsliding is minimal.

Here is an example of the Five Whys in action in the MICU and CCU central line infection study:

Problem: Lines inserted into the femoral, or groin, area are far more likely to become infected. Despite repeated admonitions and posters asking physicians to place the lines in the subclavian (shoulder) or jugular (neck) area, femoral lines continued to be placed.

1. Why did the patient have a femoral line?

   The line was inserted emergently at night.

2. Why would inserting the line at night cause a physician to choose femoral placement?

   At a teaching hospital, fellows generally end their shift at 6 PM, although several remain on call. House officers either must call a fellow in from home or insert the line themselves.

3. Why would house officers choose the femoral site?

   Because many house officers had not yet been trained to insert the subclavian lines, and femoral lines were easier and safer to insert until they were trained.

4. Why would a femoral line be left in place for four days?

   Because the risk of infection had been understated, there was little sense of urgency about removing that line and inserting a new one at a preferred site.

The real-time investigation and discipline of the Five Whys transformed central line infections from mysterious processes, in which infections were shrouded in inevitability, to recognized processes that could avert error and be improved.

In response to real-time problem solving, staff members developed a way to standardize the work. They instituted these countermeasures:

- Remove femoral lines within 12 hours and replace with a line at a preferred site.
- Replace dysfunctional catheters; do not rewire them.
- Replace lines present on transfer.
- Prefer the subclavian position for central lines. (This final countermeasure eventually led to an entire training module, complete with simulators, on which all new clinicians are trained. The money for this module and equipment came in large part from the money the hospital saved by encountering fewer central line infections.[9, 10])

product. Occasionally, as the new procedures were going into effect and sometimes thereafter, Shannon received phone calls at home from concerned nurses who had stopped a procedure. He discussed the situation with the physician in question, persuading him or her to use the proper procedure.

4. *Solve problems, one by one, as close to the time and place of occurrence as possible*. The results of the observations and real-time problem solving led the team to develop new processes and procedures together. The first four "countermeasures" or stopgaps, were adopted within 90 days: 1) remove and replace femoral lines within 12 hours; 2) replace faulty catheters rather than trying to fix (rewire) them; 3) replace central lines that patients already have when they transfer in; and 4) use the subclavian area for central line placement when possible.

Collaboratively, the MICU and CCU staffs developed protocols for line insertions and dressing changes. They standardized the line insertion kit, sterile techniques, and documentation for each procedure. Highly visible bedside displays (known as "visual

---

9. R. Shannon et al., "Economics of Central Line-Associated Bloodstream Infections," *American Journal of Medical Quality* (November/December 2006).
10. R. Shannon, D. Frndak, and N. Grunden, "Using Real-Time Problem Solving to Eliminate Central Line Infections," *Joint Commission Journal on Quality and Patient Safety* 32:9.

cues") clearly showed where the line was, and when it was inserted, eliminating time caregivers waste looking for this information.

Standardizing practices also made it easier to identify variations, when they occurred, and made it possible to mitigate their consequences before they caused infections. Weekly meetings reinforced the goal of zero infections and patient safety as a prerequisite to all work.

Since the end of the 90-day period, continued observations and real-time data gathering have led to additional learning and process improvement.

5. *Provide continuous learning for staff.* Later that year, staff noticed a small spike in the number of infections in the MICU and CCU, and discovered that the rise corresponded with the arrival of a new group of interns at this teaching hospital. Obviously, progress would have to be guarded as carefully as the patients themselves. The hospital put into place a system of instruction, including central line simulators, to ensure that all new nurses and doctors would be trained in the standardized procedures.

Results

The results of the efforts of Shannon and the care teams in the MICU and CCU were immediate, and have been sustained for three years as of this writing. The traditional approach in 2003 had yielded 49 central line infections in 37 patients, with 19 deaths, among 1,753 admissions and 1,110 lines inserted. Data from 2006 indicate three infections in three patients, with zero deaths, among 1,832 admissions and 1,898 lines inserted. Interestingly, when their illnesses were graded with the Atlas Severity Scale, the patients in 2006 (2.2) were sicker than those admitted in 2003 (1.9). See Table 2-2.

In other words, although more and sicker patients required more and more central lines during the study period, the MICU and CCU at Allegheny General Hospital sustained a greater than 95 percent reduction in central line infections in the MICU and CCU.

The units have also accrued other benefits. Because femoral line use declined, so did the time required to change dressings: from 15 minutes to

Table 2-2. Traditional vs. Perfecting Patient Care Approaches in Central Line Infections

Traditional vs. Perfecting Patient Care Approaches in Central Line Infections						
Year/ Approach	Patients with Infections	Infections	Deaths	Admissions	Lines Inserted	Atlas Severity Scale (higher score means sicker patients)
2003 Traditional approach	37	49	19	1753	1110	1.9
2006 PPC approach	3	3	0	1832	1898	2.2

5 minutes. With every line insertion and dressing, staff members save the time previously spent looking for information and equipment in each room. And as the education module on central line insertion becomes standard procedure for new doctors and nurses, infection in all intensive care units has begun to decline as well.

National spread

Progress against central line-associated bloodstream infections in the Pittsburgh region, and at Allegheny General, in particular, gained national attention. As a result, the Institute for Healthcare Improvement (IHI) made the elimination of central line-associated bloodstream infections one of the chief tenets of its 2004–2005 campaign entitled, "100,000 Lives."

• SECTION 3 •

SUSTAINING THE GAIN AGAINST CENTRAL LINE INFECTION

As mentioned in Section 2, in 2004, Dr. Richard Shannon, then-director of medicine at Allegheny General Hospital, took the Perfecting Patient Care University training and came away convinced that, by applying the principles and standardizing the work, the two intensive care units under his supervision could eliminate central line-associated bloodstream infections within 90 days.

The results of the efforts of Shannon and the care teams in the Medical Intensive Care Unit (MICU) and Coronary Care Unit (CCU) were immediate (see Section 2), and have been sustained ever since. From 2003 to 2006, despite more and sicker patients requiring more central lines, the units reduced central line infections by over 95 percent and reduced deaths to zero. Hospital leadership soon called for similar infection reduction in all its intensive care units.

In February 2007, the CCU made another landmark announcement: They had gone for one year without a single central line infection.

Making that initial gain within 90 days was one thing; sustaining and improving on it was quite another. Allegheny General has the typical dynamics of a big-city hospital; people come and go, and so do their bright initiatives. The leader of the central line-reduction effort, Dr. Shannon, accepted a position at another hospital across the state. Staff turned over as employees and new residents came and went. Given the usual hospital dynamics and the all-too-human inclination toward stasis, how did progress continue?

PHYSICIAN CHAMPION STEPS IN

As dramatic as the initial progress was against central line infection, it was not automatically self-sustaining. Because the care teams were keeping real-time data, they noticed an increase in nonstandard procedures beginning that first July, 2004—a month in which new residents arrived at this teaching hospital. Normal turnover meant new employees needed serious orientation. To keep up the progress, standardization and the culture of change had to be sustained.

In 2006, CCU Medical Director Jerome Granato, MD, was awarded a Physician Champion grant[11] by the Jewish Healthcare Foundation, PRHI's parent organization, to expand upon his year-old educational program for new nurses and residents. As part of the award, he and his team attended the Perfecting Patient Care University, and were offered occasional assistance from an on-site PRHI coach with experience in implementing these improvements.

Dr. Granato discovered that continuing to suppress central line infections meant sustaining and reinforcing the culture change through education.

"You have to make sure the improvement pot is always simmering, and the smell is always in the air," said Dr. Granato. "Everybody becomes part of an organization that defines itself as wanting to suppress central line infection."

Dr. Granato's team created an extensive online teaching module and video for residents to show them how to perform common procedures—wash hands, prepare a site, insert a central line, recognize a central line infection—the Allegheny General way. After passing a multiple choice test, they demonstrate to an instructor their newly acquired skills in a 30-minute practical session with a mannequin. This educational program has been exported to several hospitals across the United States and Canada.

Because insertion of a central line is such a common procedure, done by the youngest residents, and under a minimal amount of attending physician supervision, the payoff even for small degrees of training can be huge. Nursing new-hires also receive similar information through an online module and quiz. Both modules, for doctor and nurse, have been adopted successfully, hospital wide.

The enculturation part of the educational module is analogous to crew resource management, the airline training that inculcates the notion that every person on the crew, regardless of hierarchy, is expected to call out or

11. In early 2006, PRHI partnered the Allegheny County Medical Society and the Pennsylvania Medical Society to inaugurate the Physician Champions program. The Jewish Healthcare Foundation provided $25,000 in grants to support each of six clinical projects. All Physician Champion teams learn the principles of Perfecting Patient Care through the PRHI's Four-day University and receive on-site coaching from PRHI staff members.

stop an unsafe condition, and will not be disciplined—in fact, will be applauded—for doing so. Central line training covers all residents and nurses, and encourages any member of the care team to call out or stop non-standard procedures, with the full faith and backing of top management. The culture change, says Dr. Granato, has been revolutionary. Nurses now see themselves as the protectors and enforcers of infection control policy.

Says Dr. Granato, "Doctors travel from unit to unit; the nurses come to work in that unit every day, month, and year. Suddenly, nurses have the confidence and the authority to stop a procedure. It never used to happen, but now I might hear a nurse say, 'You know, Doctor, you're not adhering to policy. Please stop.' Or 'Doctor, this line has been in for two days. Can we take it out?' That is a revolutionary shift, and it's taken three years to create a self-sustaining environment for it."

RESULTS: ONE YEAR, NO CENTRAL LINE INFECTION

Between February 2006 and March 2007, the CCU at Allegheny General has not had one single central line infection.

"There's a little swagger among the staff," muses Dr. Granato. As part of the celebration, the hospital is making T-shirts for the CCU team that proudly proclaim The AGH CCU: "The Bug Stops Here!" See Figure 2-2.

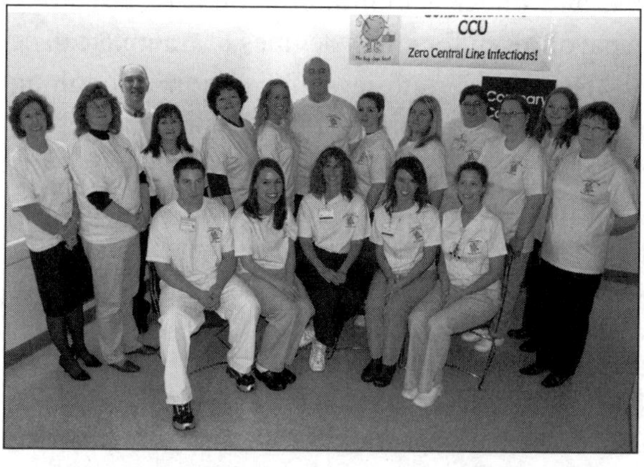

Figure 2-2. CCU nurses, physicians, infection control practitioners, and West Penn Allegheny hospital system administrators celebrate 1 year without a central line infection. Their T-shirts say, "The Bug Stops Here!"

Almost as impressive as the CCU's zero rate is the hospital-wide rate. The rate measured by the CDC's tool, the National Nosocomial Infection Surveillance System (NNIS), averages between two and seven central line infection infections per 1,000 line days, depending on the type of intensive care unit. Hospital wide, the NNIS rate at Allegheny General hovers, remarkably, between 0.9 and 1.0 per 1,000 line days.

Now, the concept of "zero infections" is extending to other hospital-acquired infections, like ventilator-associated pneumonia (VAP), antibiotic-resistant MRSA (methicillin-resistant *Staphylococcus aureus*), and urinary tract infections (UTIs).

Because VAP is "a more difficult beast"—according to Dr. Granato—harder to define and treat, the units have standardized approaches to prevent it. The standardized procedures include a rapid ventricular weaning protocol and preprinted VAP orders, which include elevating the head of the bed 30 degrees, regular tubing changes, and using chlorhexidine mouthwash twice a day. The VAP rate is down, not yet out.

Meanwhile, the central line infection work continues to expand. Through his Physician Champion work, Dr. Granato and the team are reengineering the entire process of central line insertion according to the principles of Perfecting Patient Care. Improvement has permeated the culture now, and its focus has broadened from eliminating central line infection to eliminating complications like pneumothorax (introduction of air into the pleural cavity during insertion) and arterial puncture. They are working to halve insertion time, which now stands at 45 minutes, by eliminating time lost as nurses seek missing information or tools. By streamlining and standardizing the process, Allegheny General hopes to continue to improve patient outcomes and liberate nursing time.

IMPROVEMENT IS SPREADING

Hospital culture at Allegheny General has changed for the better, with nurses more active members of the team. Dr. Granato believes that the improvements and the culture change in this one area—central line infections—made it easier to introduce improvement in other areas.

For example, the hospital now mandates that every patient undergo nasal swabbing on admission and discharge, to detect the presence of MRSA and to check its spread (see following story). It's called the active surveillance culture, and it is used in European countries that have all but eliminated the spread of MRSA.

It's one thing for hospital leadership to mandate the active surveillance culture, and another thing for the cultures to actually be taken with every patient, both on admission and discharge. In the absence of formal procedures, and in the crush of activity that surrounds admitting critically ill people or discharging them in a blizzard of prescriptions and follow-up materials, nasal swabbing is easy to skip.

Because the MICU and CCU have had formalized procedures in place for central line infections, and because the entire staff works together weekly at their Bug Meetings to discuss how to continually improve those processes, those two units have been the most successful at introducing active surveillance culturing. In the CCU, for example, about 96 percent of patients are swabbed on admission and discharge; the rest of the hospital hovers in the 80 percent range.

And the Bug Meeting focus has evolved: Three years ago, they focused on reviewing every central line infection. Now, with no more of those to review, the group is turning its attention to a one-by-one review of VAP, MRSA, and urinary tract infections (UTI).

Like his predecessor Dr. Shannon, Dr. Granato beams about the staff and its willingness to do the hard work necessary for improvement. Nevertheless, he notes, change will always be difficult.

• SECTION 4 •

REDUCING ANTIBIOTIC-RESISTANT INFECTIONS

The emergence of antibiotic-resistant organisms, such as methicillin-resistant *Staphylococcus aureus* (MRSA) has complicated the fight against hospital-acquired infections. These organisms, which defeat almost all of the antibiotics in the medical arsenal, spread through contact, usually on the hands of healthcare workers. Overuse and misuse of antibiotics are believed to exacerbate resistance,[12] as shown by the rise of distinct strains of MRSA in the community. Now ironically, community-acquired strains are also being transmitted within hospitals.

The Centers for Disease Control and Prevention (CDC) estimates that of the 90,000 people who die from hospital-acquired infections annually, 17,000 involve MRSA.[13]

"You keep hearing of high-level discussions about Anthrax, SARS and the bird flu. But MRSA is a real killer that's raging right now," says Lisa McGiffert, head of the Consumers Union campaign, Stop Hospital Infections. "If we can't stop MRSA, how could we stop a flu pandemic?"

WHAT IS MRSA AND HOW CAN IT BE STOPPED?

Although the origins of MRSA are poorly understood,[14] by the 1980s, MRSA had spread throughout the world. In the United States in 1974, just 2 percent of *Staphylococcus aureus* infections were MRSA; today, that number exceeds 60 percent.[15]

---

12. Stuart B. Levy, Antibiotic Resistance: Consequences of Inaction, Clinical Infectious Diseases, volume 33 (2001), pages S124–S129. Mayo Clinic, http://www.mayoclinic.com/health/mrsa/DS00735/ DSECTION=3.
13. As cited in ABC News Report, February 6, 2007.
14. M. C. Enright et al., "The Evolutionary History of Methicillin-Resistant *Staphylococcus aureus* (MRSA)," *Proc Natl Acad Sci U.S.* 99(11):7687–7692 (May 28, 2002).
15. C. Thronsberry NNIS. 38th ICAAC.1998; San Diego, Calif; Abstract E22; *MMWR Morb Mortal Wkly Rep*. 46:624–636 (1997). See also http://www.hospitalinfection.org/.

Active infections form only a small portion of the problem. People can be colonized with MRSA—that is, have the organism present in their bodies but show no symptoms—and spread it to others.

Stark differences in healthcare practices have led to stark differences in MRSA rates. In the Netherlands, Scandinavia, and Western Australia, where MRSA prevailed until the 1980s, it is now far less common, with sporadic outbreaks quickly contained. In Belgium and France, countries with formerly high prevalence, MRSA has been stabilized and confined.

In these countries, patients are screened on admission to the hospital to determine whether they are colonized or infected with MRSA, and then again on discharge to see whether they became colonized during their hospital stay. As previously mentioned, the technique of swabbing the nasal passages is called the active surveillance culture. If a culture is positive, that patient is isolated and, if appropriate, treated. Elective surgeries can be postponed, for example, as MRSA carriers face an increased risk of surgical site infections.

This "search and destroy" method, which relies on active surveillance cultures to screen patients, is used in Europe, but not widely in the United States. Even the most recent CDC guidelines[16] call for screening high-risk patients, not everyone, an approach criticized by advocates who insist that European countries that eradicated MRSA did so using universal screening. In one recent study, active surveillance culturing and subsequent isolation precautions resulted in a 75 percent decrease in MRSA infections in intensive care units and a 40 percent decrease elsewhere in the hospital.[17]

All people with MRSA—infected or colonized—must be isolated, and all who come in contact with them use precautions such as gloves, gowns, and masks. Any items used in the care of these patients, such as

16. Jane D. Siegel et al., "Management of Multidrug-Resistant Organisms In Healthcare Settings," U.S. Dept. of Health and Human Services, Centers for Disease Control and Prevention, Healthcare Infection Control Practices Advisory Committee, 2006. http://www.cdc.gov/ncidod/dhqp/pdf/ar/mdroGuideline2006.pdf.

17. S. Huang et al., "Impact of Routine Intensive Care Unit Surveillance Cultures and Resultant Barrier Precautions on Hospital-Wide Methicillin-Resistant Staphylococcus aureus Bacteremia," *Clinical Infectious Diseases*, Vol. 43, No. 8 (October 15, 2006).

blood pressure cuffs, thermometers, and stethoscopes, must be decontaminated or disposed of. And everyone coming into contact with patients with MRSA must practice proper hand hygiene—that is, with hand sanitizer or soap and water on entry and exit for each encounter, whether gloving or not—100 percent of the time.

PITTSBURGH'S COALITION TO ELIMINATE MRSA

In 2001, PRHI began working in conjunction with the CDC and the staff on a postsurgical unit at the Veterans' Administration Pittsburgh Health System (VAPHS), in an effort to increase compliance with procedures known to halt the spread of infection, that is, to reduce the transmission of MRSA. Statistically, the VA had a fairly low incidence of MRSA. The CDC and PRHI wanted to see how close one postsurgical unit could come to zero infections.

Healthcare workers know that hand hygiene is important to reduce the spread of pathogens that cause infection. Yet observational studies by the renowned Swiss infection control researcher, Didier Pittet, MD, show only a 10–30 percent compliance rate in practice. When hand hygiene compliance improves from just 50 percent to 75 percent, the rate of infection drops by half.[18] The pilot work at 4 West, an inpatient surgery unit at the confluence of 12 surgery lines, would find new ways to encourage compliance with hand hygiene and other known, agreed-upon guidelines to protect patients from infection.

The VA Pittsburgh's top leadership joined with the CDC in making the necessary resources available to create this pilot program on 4 West—resources that included the full-time service of a respected nurse leader, Ellesha McCray, MSN, RN, to help lead the effort. Although confined to a unit, the effort marked a new level of collaboration among government agencies, community-based PRHI, and frontline caregivers.

---

18. "Summaries for Patients, Hand-Washing Practices and Beliefs of Physicians," *Annals of Internal Medicine*, Vol 141:1, I–38.

APPLICATION IN A SMALL SETTING

Applying Perfecting Patient Care principles in such a limited way—on one unit, against one microorganism—initially troubled the on-site coach that PRHI assigned. Peter Perreiah, an engineer who learned the Toyota system through his years at Alcoa, spoke the language of cultural change and institution-wide transformation. Although organizations like Alcoa and Toyota use these principles throughout their organizations—"wall to wall"—Perreiah also had experience applying them in small settings. Nevertheless, Toyota "purists" may have blanched at applying the techniques so narrowly.

Eventually, the cascade of improvements that followed—from improving access to supplies, to cleaning wheelchairs—could not be confined to a single unit and soon proliferated throughout the organization. Most important, the improvements provided staff with more time to devote to prevention, like 100 percent hand hygiene and adherence to isolation precautions.

"The first thing we had to do was change the question," said Perreiah. "We had to stop asking, 'Why *don't* you follow procedures?' and start asking 'Why *can't* you follow procedures?' Workers often confront multiple barriers that prevent them from getting something done. It's a principle in Perfecting Patient Care that you follow those reasons: Ask WHY five times and you'll usually uncover the root cause."

Perreiah and McCray set the goal high: *4 West would strive to create an ideal system where each patient receives what is needed on demand, without waste or defect, one by one, immediately. For the worker, waste will be eliminated; the environment will be physically, emotionally, professionally safe; and work will be redesigned and balanced so that hand hygiene and other precautions would be built right in to the way work is done.*

DESCRIBING THE CURRENT CONDITION

But they had to start somewhere. So they started by collecting two key pieces of data that would help reveal problems in their true dimension:

1. *Which patients were infected or colonized with MRSA?* The pilot program required and paid for nasal swabbing (active surveillance

cultures) for all patients on admission and discharge from 4 West. This procedure produced something close to "real-time" data, letting staff know who needed to be isolated on admission, and whether a patient had been colonized or infected during hospitalization.

"The ability to say, 'You remember Mr. Smith, who was released last week? Well, when he came in, he didn't have MRSA, but when he left, he'd been colonized.' You say that to a professional, and that one data point has far more impact than retrospective quarterly data on infection 'rates,'" said Perreiah.

2. *How often did staff use appropriate standard and contact precautions?* Standard precautions include hand hygiene on entry and exit from a room for patients who do not have MRSA, and gowning and gloving when there is a risk of exposure to bodily fluids. Contact precautions require hand hygiene and personal protective equipment (PPE) like gloves, gowns, hats, and masks for all healthcare workers who approach patients in isolation for MRSA or other communicable diseases.

   The team created an observation checklist and trained several staff members to observe hand hygiene and PPE compliance consistently. Observation is not a superficial exercise. The team performed over 1,000 of them over two years, to establish data on how often people performed adequate hand hygiene, and whether or not behavior was changing. In the beginning, hand hygiene compliance fell in the range of 50 percent, in line with other observational studies.

COUNT ON RUNNING OUT

It didn't take long to discover one reason why workers were having trouble complying with infection-control procedures. Some glove dispensers were empty. Some rooms had gowns; some did not. Not every room had an alcohol hand rub dispenser in a consistent, convenient location. Every day, staff could count on running out of something. Perreiah and McCray began to look for ways to stabilize the system.

Workers on 4 West first established: (1) who would be responsible for restocking gloves and gowns (the nurse's assistant); (2) how often supplies would be checked (daily); and (3) how the cupboards would be labeled so that any deficiency would immediately become obvious (see Figures 2-3, 2-4, and 2-5). The notification system was decidedly low-tech—color-coded construction paper taped to the back of the cabinets, with pink designating the nurse's assistant, blue the technician, and so forth. The system was based on "pull," that is, stock was replenished only when it reached a trigger level. This eliminated the syndrome of too much of one thing, not enough of another.

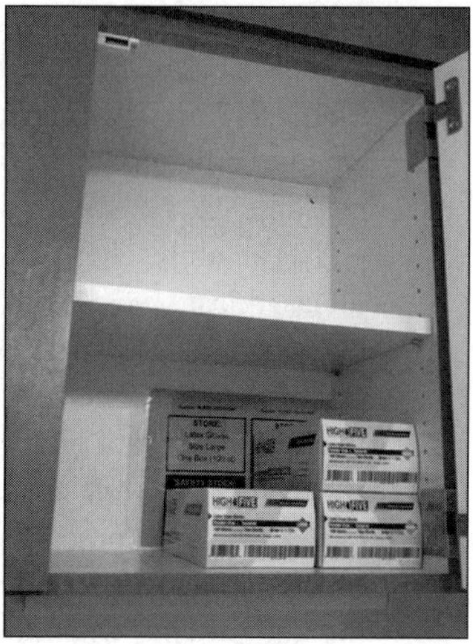

Figure 2-3. Color-coded posters on the back of cupboards clearly show when the glove supply is low, and indicate who is responsible for replenishing it.

"The cupboards talk to us now," said McCray. "We can't be out of something and not know it."

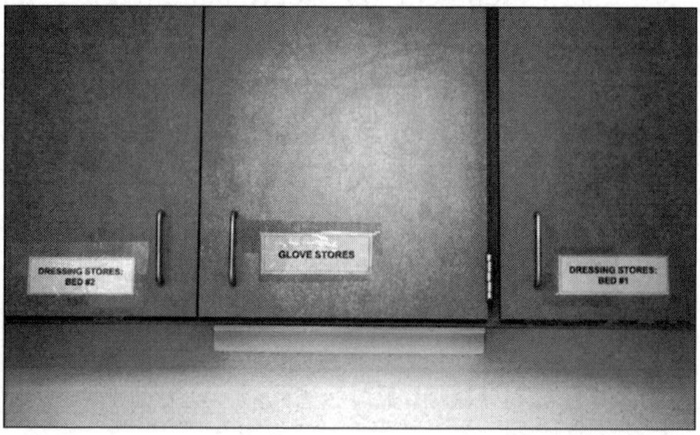

Figure 2-4. No more opening and closing of cupboards to find the right thing. All entry rooms are equipped the same way, and signs are visible.

Within days, the new system became successful: "Stashes" of gloves and gowns workers had secreted away came out of closets as the system began to support the workers. Within weeks, the new supply system was introduced throughout the floor. Interestingly, although gloving compliance went up, glove consumption and costs dropped by about 15 percent. Those "stashes" had been costly.

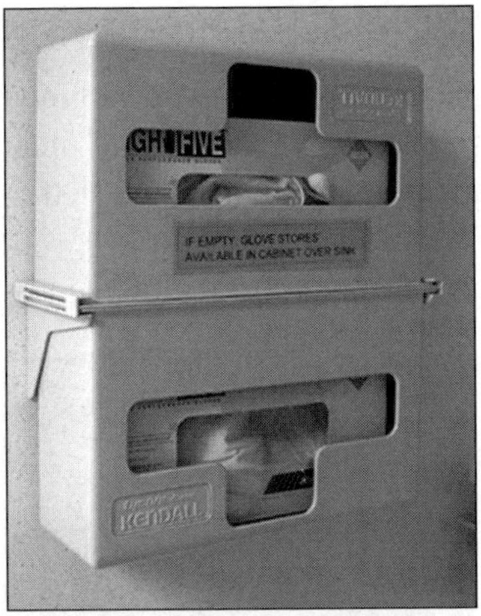

Figure 2-5. Glove boxes with two sizes of gloves are hung in a convenient place in every room now. Signage shows where to get more if one is empty.

Gowns were bulky, uncomfortable and scarce. The team experimented by ordering different gowns until the staff agreed upon a style that was easy to store and use. With always enough comfortable, disposable gowns at the ready, reasons for not wearing them evaporated. Because they had been part of the decision, staff members wore the gowns.

In one instance, a question arose about gowning: When entering a patient's room for an encounter that would not require contact—such as saying, "Good Morning," or asking a question—would it be necessary to gown? To deal with this eventuality, the team taped off a one-foot square floor area just inside the room. This unequivocal visual cue, borrowed directly from the factory floor, tells employees that they may enter but may not go past the line without gowning. (See Figure 2–6.)

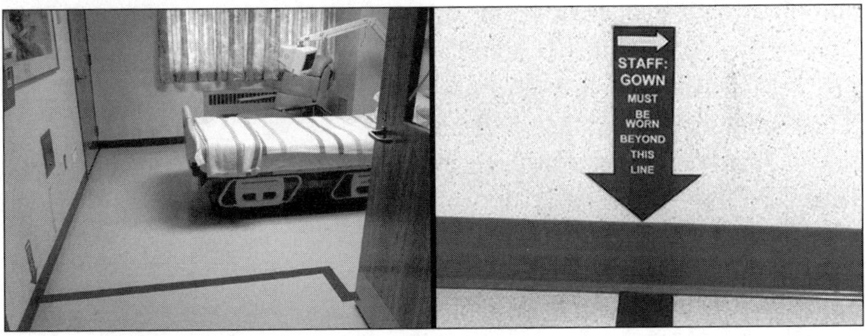

Figure 2-6. *Straight from the factory floor*: Arrows and lines on the floor unequivocally show staffers how far they may come into the room before they must glove and gown. Some studies showed that patients in isolation may see less of the nursing staff, and that the requirement to glove and gown on entry to the room makes it harder for nurses to look in with a routine, "Good morning, Mr. Smith." With lines on the floor, staff members are free to check in on a patient frequently, and need to glove and gown only when going past the line. No matter what, though, hand hygiene is practiced on entry and exit from every room.

DEDICATED EQUIPMENT, STANDARDIZED CLEANING

Patients who harbor MRSA must be isolated. The stethoscopes, blood pressure cuffs, and other medical devices must not be shared with other patients. When a physician examines a patient in isolation, which stethoscope is used?

Ideally, commonly used items are stored, cleaned, and kept in the isolation room. But too often, there was no stethoscope at the ready. The improvement team decided to place hot pink stethoscopes in the isolation rooms. The color coding served two purposes: to mark the instrument as one strictly for the isolation room; and to keep the physician from accidentally walking off with it. (See Figure 2-7.)

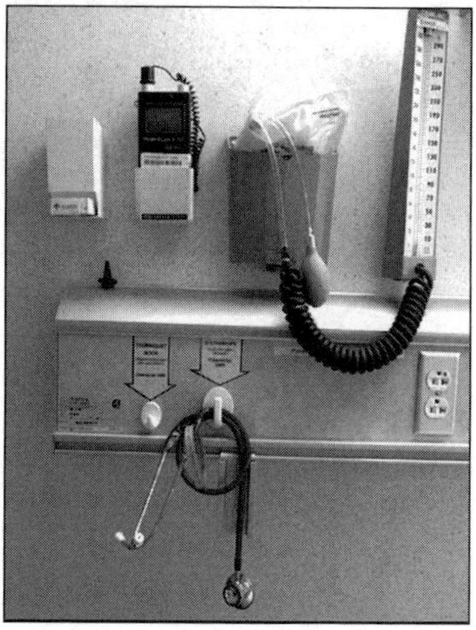

Figure 2-7. Color-coded equipment and signs mean equipment stays in isolation rooms.

Cleaning of the rooms was also standardized. Working with housekeeping staffers, the improvement team devised a standard way to clean an isolation room and everything in it, complete with checklist. If an infection or colonization occurred, the problem-solving team could understand whether a nonstandard cleaning practice had contributed to the problem. Before, this information would have been lost.

FINDING TIME

The most frequent reason given for skipping hygiene precautions was "lack of time." Workers feel tremendous pressure to complete their work in a system that does not ensure that they have what they need, when they need it. Setting up a system to guarantee a steady supply of gloves and gowns helped workers recoup several minutes of work time each day, and immediately raised compliance rates.

Workers are often instructed to "find the time" to do important tasks. McCray and Perreiah did not set their sights on adding more work to be completed in the same amount of time. Instead, they looked for ways to actually find time for workers by eliminating tasks they didn't or shouldn't have to do (waste).

5S HELPS WORKERS FIND MORE TIME

Perreiah and McCray introduced a relatively simple, rapid, low-cost, low-tech way of finding even more time for workers. It's called 5S, which is shorthand for Sort, Set in order, Shine, Standardize, and Sustain. It's an American idea exported to Japan after World War II, now reimported with a Japanese, people-centered philosophy attached.

Before World War II, many American businesses had codified the idea that a clean workplace is a productive workplace. As Americans helped the Japanese reconstruct their industries after the war, they found the Japanese to be ready students.

Before long, the Western idea of the orderly and productive workplace became tied to the Eastern idea of respect for the worker's well-being and morale. Out of this blend of philosophies came a technique for creating the orderly workplace; a technique directed not by a distant manager, but by the esteemed worker.

The name, 5S, refers to a sequence of steps that translate approximately as follows:

- *Sort.* Remove all items from the workplace that are not needed for current operations. A crowded workplace is hard to work in and costly to maintain.
- *Set in order.* Arrange needed items so that they are easy to use. Label them so that they're easy to find, clean, and put away. This degree of order improves communication and reduces the frustration of wasted time and motion.
- *Shine.* Clean the floors, walls, and equipment. When things are kept in top condition, when someone needs to use something, it is always ready. In a hospital environment, cleanliness is extremely important to staff member and patient alike.

- *Standardize.* By integrating the first three steps into everyday work, the continuous restoration of order is built into work routines. "Backsliding" stops.
- *Sustain.* This involves exercising leadership to keep morale high about preserving workplace order. If the rewards for keeping order outweigh the rewards for going back to the old way of doing things, people will make orderliness a habit.

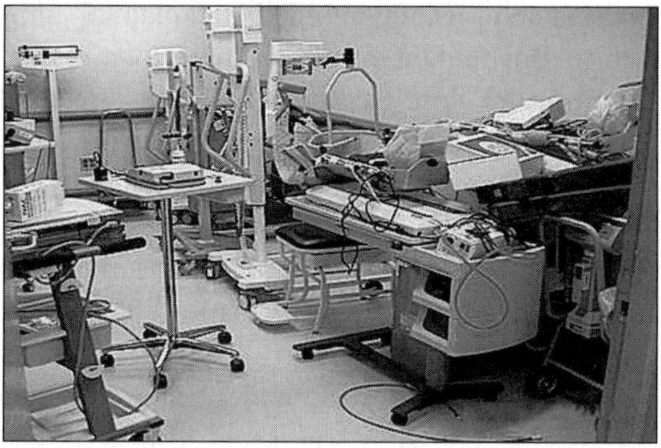

Figure 2-8. Equipment storage room: before. Like in many American hospitals, a mix of equipment, not easy to retrieve.

The process got started on 4 West when workers took a long, honest look at their Equipment Storage Room. It looked like a typical storage room in any American hospital—a mix of often- and seldom-used equipment, stored in no particular order (Figure 2-8.). It took time to find equipment, and it was difficult to walk around in the room. Items relying on recharged batteries were not always plugged in. It wasn't clear where or in what condition things were supposed to be stored.

More to the point: Were they cleaned before or after use? Were they unintended vectors of infection?

Following a deliberate process over a few weeks (Figure 2-9), staff members on 4 West reduced the inventory in the room, while still maintaining access to what they needed when they needed it. About $20,000 worth of seldom-used equipment was released for use in other areas of the hospital.

Now, signs clearly denote where each piece of equipment is to be stored, how it is to be cleaned, whether or not it is to be plugged in, etc. The visual cues leave no doubt about the expectations. Anyone can walk into the room, find equipment, and recognize what is already checked out—

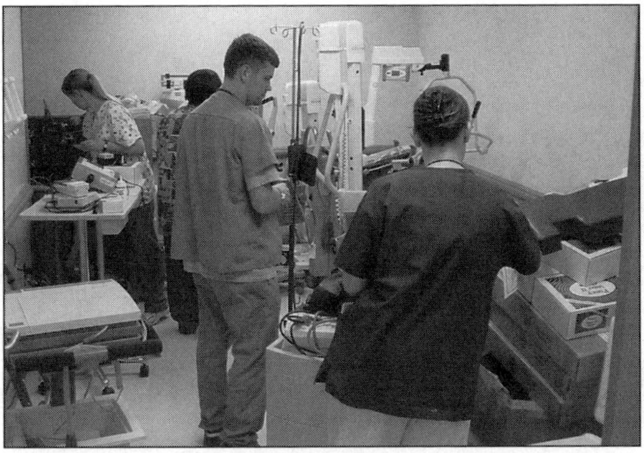

Figure 2-9. Over several days, employees 5S the equipment room, sorting, standardizing, cleaning—and sometimes removing—equipment.

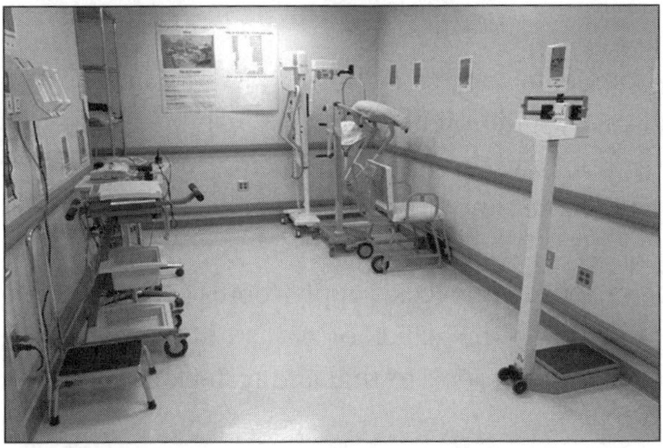

Figure 2-10. *After*: Equipment is always clean, easy to find, plugged in, and charged up. Posters above each piece of equipment shows exactly where it goes. A larger poster on the rear wall shows the "before" picture, congratulating and encouraging the workers on their progress.

whether it has been cleaned, and so forth. (See Figure 2-10.)

In the three years since the incorporation of 5S improvements, the room and equipment have been maintained in sparkling clean condition with little problem. Since cleaning is built into the work itself, backsliding is minimal.

The Equipment Storage Room worked so well that staffers on other units soon learned 5S. In short order, units on the fifth and sixth floors organized their storage rooms according to the principles. Soon, the Clean Supply Rooms followed suit, looking now more like organized, ergonomically correct retail stores, rather than the chaotic environment that once prevailed. (See Figure 2-11.)

"Who could be against this? Having the storage areas orderly like this really saves time and frustration. It's better for patients," said Shedale Pinnix-Tindall, nurse manager on 6 West, who adopted 5S on that unit. "Besides, it's so much easier to keep it this way."

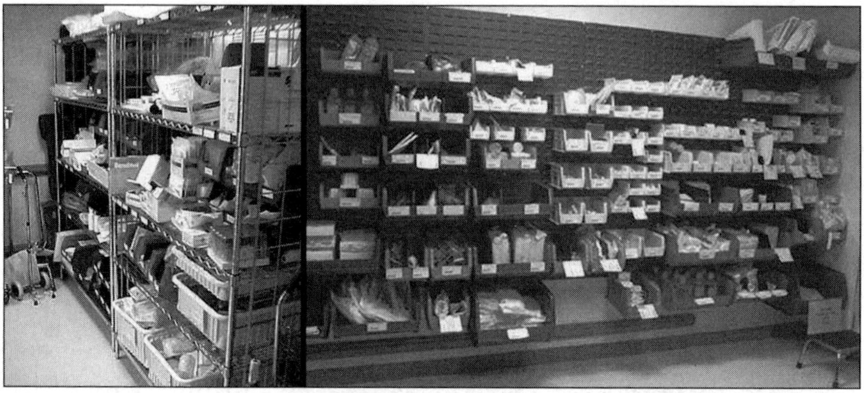

Figure 2-11. *Left*, the Clean Supply Room was disorganized. It took technicians up to 30 minutes to restock, and took nurses several steps and minutes to obtain materials for a routine blood draw. *Right*, the room is now organized, color-coded by the type of procedure. Blood draw equipment is in one spot, right by the door. Technicians can restock in just 5 minutes.

John R. Finkley, environmental aide said, "Since we did 5S on 4 West, we can get what we need easily and quickly for every patient. There's no guessing. You just open the door and go right to the item. I spend less time cleaning that room, so I have more time to clean every piece of equipment thoroughly."

Soon, at the behest of various employees, supply rooms across the hospital also underwent 5S, freeing up thousands of dollars in unused items, and dramatically reducing the time it took to find and restock supplies.

THE AWKWARD CONVERSATION: *DID YOU WASH YOUR HANDS?*

Harvard professor, Lucian Leape, MD, commonly called the father of the modern healthcare quality-improvement movement in the United States, has defined organizational culture as "the way we do things around here."

Creating a culture that would reinforce 100 percent hand hygiene was not easy. It's well known that failure of hand hygiene puts patients at risk for acquiring infections. Yet healthcare workers usually hesitate to call out hand hygiene lapses on the part of their colleagues.

McCray uses the analogy that if your neighbor runs a stop sign up the block, you'll probably have a word with him or her. Skipping hand hygiene is so serious for patients that the same instinctive reaction needs to occur.

"We're surrounding the problem," says McCray. "We're thinking systematically about how to remove the barriers that keep workers from performing hand hygiene every time."

After reviewing observational data showing low compliance, particularly among physicians, the chiefs of staff and surgery concluded that policies needed to support better habits. Their new rule required 100 percent hand hygiene on entry and exit from a patient's room.

Alcohol rub dispensers had been installed, but were rarely used, because of misperceptions about them. Some workers thought soap and water a superior method of hand sanitization; others found the alcohol drying to the hands. Alcohol rub is recommended by the CDC as superior to hand washing in certain situations. To reinforce the preference for alcohol rub, the improvement team prominently displayed a poster at the VAPHS. This key visual cue demonstrates to workers how well the alcohol rub works (Figure 2–12).

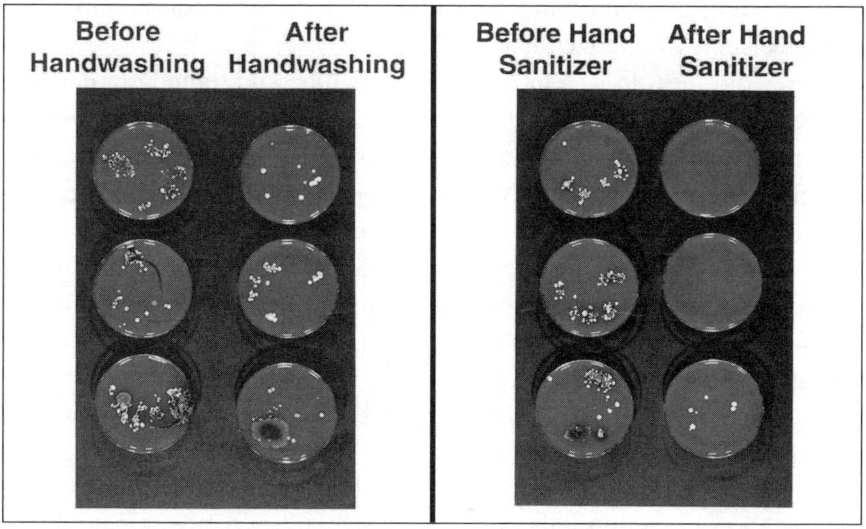

Figure 2–12. The hands of in-house physicians were cultured before and after handwashing, then before and after using hand sanitizer. The posters were placed throughout the hospital to reinforce the CDC preference for alcohol hand sanitizer for routine encounters (not involving bodily fluids). Use of sanitizer increased.

When some workers complained that the alcohol gel dried their hands, other types of alcohol-based products were tried. Workers seemed satisfied with a foam product. Not only did it save time over soap and water, and in most cases work better, data showed that those who used the alcohol-based foam actually improved the condition of their skin. Those data were posted in employee areas along with other improvement data. Compliance went up.

McCray followed up with 4 West staffers conducting continuous training about the risks and benefits of hand hygiene. "We don't talk so much about policies," said McCray, "but more about what you need to do to protect the patient. When you address the problem in real life, people get it much more quickly. We ask people to sanitize their hands on entry and exit of all rooms, to establish the habit."

Nobody wants to tell someone or be told to wash their hands. The traditional occupational hierarchy of a hospital creates great discomfort for people who want to remind others about hand hygiene.

"We were able to create an environment in 4 West that spread throughout the hospital," said McCray. "A person's job title no longer gets in the way of doing the right thing for patients. I have seen nurses reminding chief residents to sanitize their hands."

How did they do it? McCray gave staff time and training to devise a prepared script to use when they saw somebody take a hygiene shortcut (see sidebar). McCray and others began using the script themselves, as a signal to others that it was safe—and expected—for them to do so. The team created posters, featuring respected hospital leaders giving a "high sign" to encourage hand hygiene. Soon after the posters began to appear, workers began to raise their hands to signify to one another that this was a time for hand hygiene. Hand hygiene compliance, as measured by soap and alcohol rub utilization, went up in the wake of this campaign.

Creating what McCray calls a "global culture change" also involved the patients. Signs were designed by a team from patient care services and housekeeping to inform patients of their right to be treated with clean hands. Large, prominent signs urge patients to speak out. McCray recounts, "One doctor tells his students about the time a patient stopped him. He says, 'The first time a patient reminds you to wash your hands, you'll never forget it.'"

Preparing for the Awkward Conversation

Training included the hows and whys of that awkward conversation, calling out lapses in hand hygiene on the part of coworkers. The module includes an actual script, which many staff members carry on a card in their pockets. The following is an excerpt from the VAPHS training module on MRSA reduction, which is available online at http://www.va.gov/Pittsburgh/mrsa/index.htm.

Script: *"Excuse me. I thought I saw you exit that patient room without performing hand hygiene. This hospital requires all of us to perform hand hygiene when entering and exiting a room."*

Support your fellow healthcare workers in complying with precautions. Constant pressure from everyone can break bad habits and form good ones.

Do's

- Act as soon as you see a violation.
- Be graceful.
- Accept comments gracefully.
- Be brief.

Don'ts

- Don't embarrass.
- Don't lecture.
- Don't argue.
- Don't threaten or ridicule.

Figure 2-13 may look complicated, but it is worth studying. The 4-West nurses came to know this chart, which connects their infection control efforts with patient outcomes. The top line depicts the level of MRSA that exists generally in the population: Patients who are colonized or infected on admission. The bottom line shows the rate of transmission (colonization and infection) in the hospital.

One would expect that the more MRSA exists in the general population, the higher the "pressure" for its spread within the hospital if precautions are not always followed. At the left of the chart, in January, at the beginning of the intervention, the parallel gray arrows show exactly such a correlation.

But look what happens around May. The countermeasures are taking effect, and even as the MRSA pressure increases (more people are being

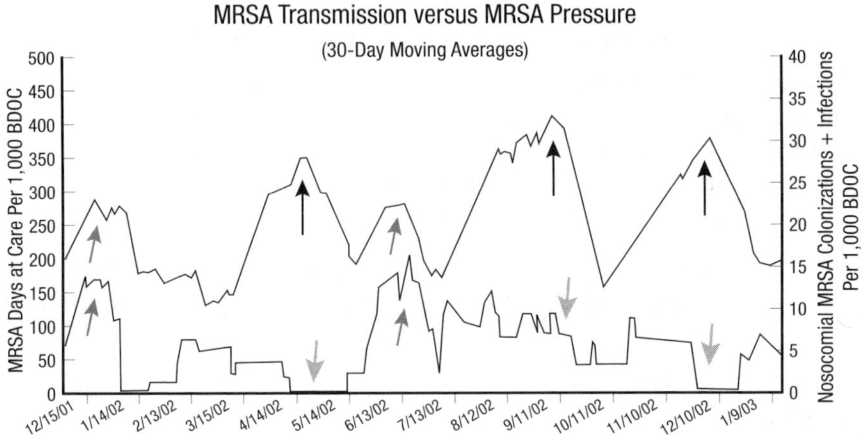

Figure 2-13. This chart demonstrates the decreased rate of transmission that occurred using new hand-washing procedures, despite an increased level of MRSA.

admitted who are colonized or infected), fewer in-hospital transmissions occur. This relationship is noted by black and white arrows.

In July, there's a brief reversion, where higher pressure results again in more MRSA transmission. That period of time corresponded to an unusually high staff turnover, requiring that nurses from other floors, where the intense hand hygiene and other countermeasures had not yet been done, filled about 60 percent of the day-to-day staffing.

Once staffing issues were resolved in September, and all staff was consistently trained in the countermeasures, MRSA transmission again declined, regardless of the notable MRSA pressure in November and January.

MRSA PROJECT TODAY

From its status as a "pilot program" on 4 West, the VA MRSA project has grown to encompass all 17 VA hospitals across Pennsylvania, and was recently rolled out in all 150 VA hospitals nationwide. Using the Toyota-based techniques adapted by Perreiah and McCray, these hospitals now require active surveillance cultures for MRSA on all patients at admission, transfer, and discharge. The effort stands at the forefront of the national effort to eradicate MRSA in the United States. In addition to reducing morbidity and mortality among patients, the VA believes that testing all patients (about $8 per patient) will ultimately cost less than treating MRSA infections (estimated at $25,000 to $50,000 per patient).

As a result of the screening, each participating hospital will know its current MRSA rate. Patients can be isolated, and especially where Perfecting Patient Care has been acculturated, healthcare workers now have the systems to enable them to take contact precautions 100 percent of the time when caring for their patients, reducing the chance of infection and transmission.

• SECTION 5 •

REDESIGNING A SYSTEM: THE WHEELCHAIRS

One of the more haunting aspects of Steve Lares' story in Chapter 1 involves his suffering while the staff at a major urban hospital struggled for half an hour to find a wheelchair. Staff members at every hospital meet the issue of wheelchair availability with negative emotions: It takes time to find one. Sometimes it's not the kind of wheelchair the patient needs. Sometimes it isn't even clean.

For the team on 4 West trying to find time for workers and stop the transmission of MRSA, the wheelchair system became a problem. But getting clean wheelchairs quickly on 4 West required a system-wide solution. The problem came to light because so many veterans were late getting to and from their physical therapy appointments. With the physical therapy department chronically bottlenecked, workers there were frustrated, too.

The staff asked, *"Why can't we provide clean wheelchairs in the time and place needed, in the configuration that the patient needs?"*

A little investigation revealed that wheelchairs were a big system problem. How quickly a patient in need can receive a wheelchair says a lot about how the whole system is working, akin to trains running on time. Under the leadership of Peter Perreiah and Ellesha McCray, Perfecting Patient Care techniques were about to spread throughout the entire VA Pittsburgh system.

From 4 West, observations and problem solving extended to all three of the VA's Pittsburgh locations: the acute-care hospital; the H.J. Heinz long-term care facility; and the psychiatric facility.

The wheelchair problem had three components: 1) supply, having enough wheelchairs when and where needed; 2) fit, having a wheelchair of proper size and configuration; and 3) cleanliness, ensuring that the wheelchairs are in a condition unlikely to transfer contaminants.

PROBLEM: NOT JUST ANY WHEELCHAIR

A correct wheelchair constitutes more than a matter of comfort: It can affect patient health and safety. Getting patients out of bed safely and maintaining their physical activity using wheelchairs is important in reducing the risk of respiratory and urinary tract infections, as well as improving a patient's mental outlook.

Understanding individual patient needs is the first step in improving physical activity. Larger patients require wider wheelchairs. Diabetic patients often need wheelchairs with leg rests to protect their vulnerable feet. Patients undergoing hip replacement need wheelchairs with reclining backs to avoid postoperative dislocation, while cancer patients may require smaller wheelchairs.

At the H.J. Heinz long-term care facility, patients require wheelchairs in which they can sit comfortably for several hours: Wheelchairs with substantial padding and high backs, again in various sizes (Figure 2-14). Quick-release seat belts prevent patients from falling out of wheelchairs, and antitipping devices prevent the chairs from tumbling backward. Altogether, the VA system requires wheelchairs of about a dozen different configurations.

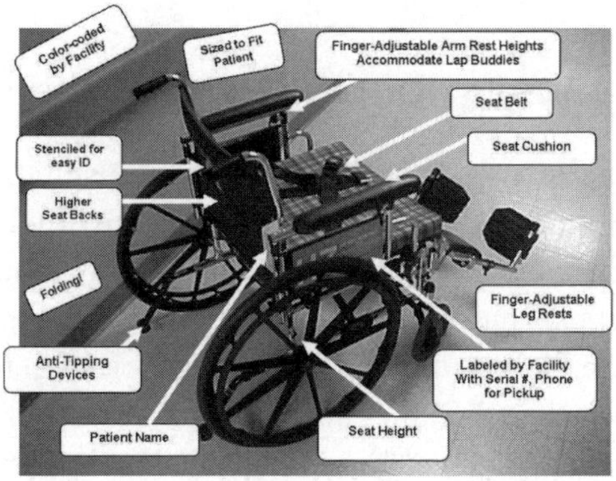

Figure 2-14. The VA's investment in new wheelchairs stabilized a chronic system shortage. The new chairs are color-coded by facility. The diagram shows the special, patient–centered features of the most intensively used wheelchairs in the system, those at the Heinz long-term care facility.

PROBLEM: SUPPLY AND DEMAND

On an average day, the postsurgical 4 West unit serves about 25 patients. Yet on average, those patients need transportation to more than 40 appointments—from physical therapy to imaging to hemodialysis. At most hospitals, wheelchairs are shared equipment, and that sharing can create long waits or searching. Too often, patients arrived late to appointments across the hospital, creating delays (lost and wasted hours) across the entire hospital system.

PROBLEM: HIDING AND HOARDING

At hospitals everywhere, hiding and hoarding are common behavior. When the system does not supply what is needed when it's needed, people learn to distrust the system. In a heroic attempt to provide the patients with what they need, staff members sometimes stash wheelchairs in closets, bathrooms, or empty rooms, where they can't be seen and used by others. The problem is, even if enough wheelchairs exist in a hospital, hoarding can create a wheelchair shortage.

OBSERVATION: INVENTORY

One example, at the acute-care hospital, typified the problem: Of five reclining wheelchairs purchased just months earlier, only one remained. With some sleuthing, the problem-solving team discovered that, when patients had been transferred from the acute-care hospital to the long-term care facility, they had been transported in the reclining wheelchairs, which then stayed on the receiving end. As a result, both the long-term care facility and psychiatric hospitals had a plethora of wheelchairs that were, generally, the wrong kind for their patients. Their problem was finding storage for the unwanted wheelchairs because no system was in place to return wheelchairs to the acute-care hospital.

EXPERIMENTING WITH SUPPLY SOLUTIONS

But how could healthcare workers know which wheelchair belongs where? After cleaning all of the chairs in the system, the problem solvers had associated unique wheelchair colors with each facility by applying labels on the side panels and stenciling the seat backs. In this way, whenever a stray wheelchair was spotted on a unit, healthcare workers would immediately know if it needed to be returned to its home facility.

The problem-solving team next identified convenient public places for wheelchairs to be placed between uses. At the acute-care hospital, the group studied the hospital layout, identifying traffic patterns, congregating areas, and so on. They worked with people in every unit, from inpatient nursing to nuclear medicine, to define the best places to locate wheelchairs. Together they designated 30 convenient Wheelchair Courtesy Points throughout the hospitals. The most significant stores are near the main entrance, in a large elevator lobby and in a recreation room. Escorts now return wheelchairs to the forward staging areas in a predictable pattern. At all facilities, wheelchairs from transferred patients are cleaned and collected at transfer points near the loading docks. Twice a week, a truck that brings supplies also returns wheelchairs to their home facilities.

At the long-term care facility, physical therapists assess patients' wheelchair needs within 24 hours of arrival and issue appropriately configured chairs to meet their individual needs. When a patient is discharged, members of the housekeeping staff clean the wheelchair, and mechanics check it and return it to Physical Therapy for reissue.

The VA did make a one-time, substantial investment in new wheelchairs to have the number and variety of wheelchairs meet the needs of long-term patients. However, in the three years since the system was deployed, data show that the recirculation system and Wheelchair Courtesy Points are working. More patients are on time for their appointments, and less-quantifiable outcomes, such as patient comfort and worker satisfaction, also have improved. Finally, the clear VA identification on the wheelchairs quickly paid off: Within weeks, dozens of chairs were returned to the hospital that would have been lost from the VA system in the past.

EXPERIMENTING WITH CLEANING

Presenting clean wheelchairs to staff and patients is important. The group hit upon the idea of using a cart washer in another area of the hospital to clean the wheelchairs thoroughly. The cart washers (enclosed units similar to dishwashers) use high-pressure hot water to "detail" the chairs. During off hours, the wheelchairs were processed one by one, and in 12 days, the whole fleet had been washed.

The effect was dazzling—wheelchairs that looked brand new.

Borrowing washers from another unit wasn't viewed as a long-term solution. It was daunting to trek a hundred-plus wheelchairs to one place in the hospital. Instead, the team tried a portable cart-washing unit capable of turning out a clean wheelchair every 4 minutes. A portable washer could be moved to the wheelchairs, instead of vice versa. In the end, two portable cart washers serviced the entire wheelchair fleet. One is housed at the main University Drive hospital; the other is at the Heinz long-term care facility.

In some units, plumbing was readily available. In others, a simple plumbing retrofit met the need. The procedure began to work; the group called ahead of time, giving the unit advance notice that the cart washer would be available on-site. Two-person teams did the work, with one retrieving chairs and one monitoring the wash cycle.

At University Drive, the group quickly discovered that the optimal time for cleaning the chairs was during the evenings. When the clinics were closed, there were fewer calls for wheelchairs, and the hospital was less congested.

Within several days of the cart washer's arrival, each of the over 200 wheelchairs at the Heinz long-term care facility was cleaned. Residents at the facility spend most of their days in the wheelchairs, so frequent cleaning and maintenance is a must for patients' comfort and well-being.

The housekeeping staff at Heinz established a monthly schedule for washing and inspecting every wheelchair. The housekeeping staff also formalized procedures for urgent need. When a wheelchair needed immediate attention, the housekeeping staff came promptly to clean it.

Staff members at each hospital have now developed cleaning patterns based on patient usage. For example, at Heinz, where long-term care patients virtually "live" in their wheelchairs for hours each day, cleaning is more frequent. At University Drive, the cleaning schedule accommodates acute-care patients who use wheelchairs, intermittently, for transport between units.

CONFUSING THE ARTIFACT WITH THE SYSTEM

Staff from other hospitals have visited the VA and have made positive remarks on the Wheelchair Courtesy Points (Figure 2–15). Confusing the artifact with the system, many hurriedly returned to their hospitals to establish Wheelchair Courtesy Points. However, they were disappointed when wheelchairs continued to disappear, or show up without having been

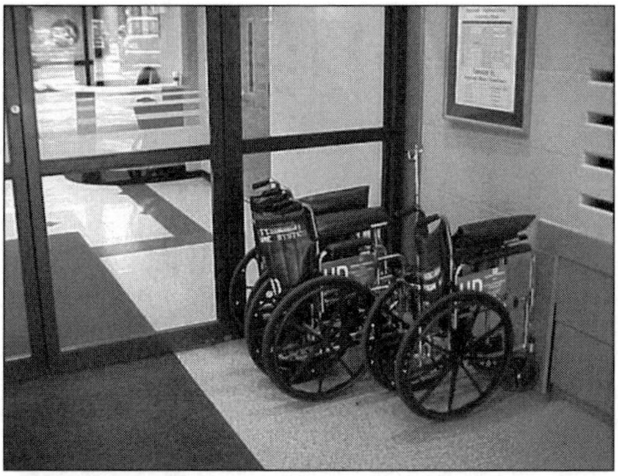

Figure 2-15. By the front door of the VA is one of several wheelchair courtesy areas, where wheelchairs are always available. Underlying this seemingly simple innovation was a year's worth of work to ensure a self-sustaining system of wheelchairs of the proper size, configuration, and cleanliness were always available.

cleaned. Without the underlying system, the signs, charts, and visual cues cannot create change.

"SIDE EFFECT" OF WHEELCHAIR PROGRAM

Solving the wheelchair problem meant less time wasted by couriers, but also more veterans making their physical therapy appointments on time. Fewer cancellations meant better utilization of staff and resources in the physical therapy department (Figure 2-16).

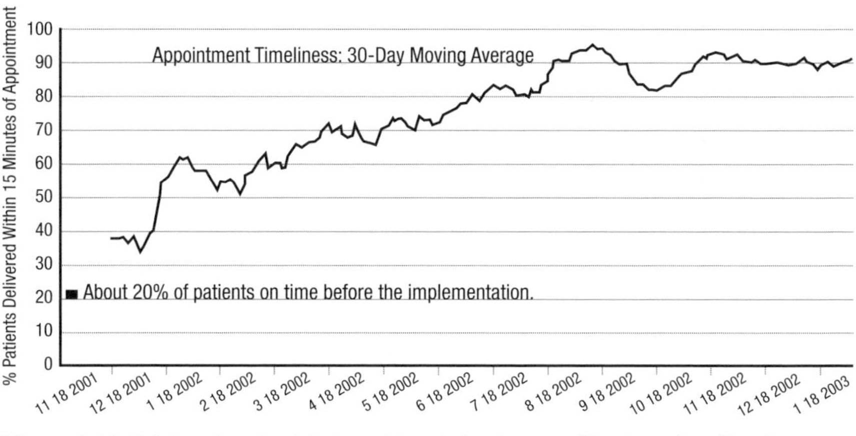

Figure 2-16. Solving the wheelchair problem led to better utilization of staff and resources in the physical therapy department.

CHAPTER 3

Moving Closer to the Patient

CASE STUDIES

- **Section 1. Housekeepers: key to reducing injuries and infections.** When a 20-year veteran housekeeper developed occasional backaches, the hospital looked to process improvement to fix the problem. In the process, the hospital looked to systemic improvement.
- **Section 2. Putting nurses in the driver's seat.** Giving nurses standardized ways to respond immediately to certain emergencies makes patients safer and nurses more satisfied.
- **Section 3. Stopping the revolving door on nursing turnover.** A nurse-led program stopped the exodus of nurses in a liver transplant unit, bringing turnover from 12 percent to zero in a year.

PRHI was invited into various organizations over the years to observe and suggest ways to make improvements. Sometimes, employees in an area of the hospital had read about the Perfecting Patient Care improvements made elsewhere and wanted to try them out.

Three barriers often led to frustration:

1. Unless top management supports and desires a transformational change in the way work is done across the institution, the effort will not get far. Even efforts designed to be confined to one unit naturally must spread to other units (i.e., admitting, lab, pharmacy, wheelchairs) if improvement is to happen. For spread to occur, top management and clinical leaders must support change.
2. Enthusiastic employees, while a key to progress, must be supported with education and training in the methods before implementing changes.

3. A high level of turnover among healthcare professionals—over 5 percent in Pennsylvania—makes continuity of improvements, not to mention continuity of care, difficult.

Healthcare institutions face enormous financial challenges, and it is understandable that many of them want to begin with cost-cutting. However, the Toyota-based philosophy relies first and foremost on respect for the customer and the employee—not on saving money. In a hospital setting, this respect extends to patients and employees (people). Where top management shows respect by helping employees redesign the way work is done, and where employees are given the tools and training to accomplish this work, progress occurs. (And financial savings follow.)

The stories in this chapter demonstrate that, when every employee is respected in the workplace—intellectually, emotionally, and physically—creativity blossoms, and solutions pour forth. Systems improve, patients and employees are safer, and staff turnover can be reversed. Financial savings are a natural consequence of work redesign.

• SECTION 1 •

HOUSEKEEPERS: KEY TO REDUCING INJURIES AND INFECTIONS

Hospital leaders across Southwestern Pennsylvania occasionally invite PRHI staff to visit their hospitals and help them spot ways to accelerate improvements. When Dave Martin, president and CEO of UPMC St. Margaret, made such a request in early 2004, PRHI on-site coach Debra Thompson, MSN, RN, paid a visit. Thompson teaches the basics of Perfecting Patient Care to leaders expressing interest.

"Where to begin always seems to be a challenge. It can seem overwhelming. But we've found that everyone can agree on one thing: They want a clean hospital," said Thompson.

With that in mind, Thompson, Martin, Environmental Services Director John Merkt, and other hospital leaders set off to the floors, where the work is done, to begin detailed observations of hand hygiene.

Were staff members sanitizing their hands on entry to and exit from every room, every time? If not, what were the barriers? Were soap and alcohol rub dispensers easily accessible? Were they always full? Were gloves always available, and did staff use them appropriately?

Into the patient's domain

These observations soon moved directly into patient rooms, and the questions expanded. Housekeeping staff were among the most observant when it came to hand hygiene, but they seemed frantically busy.

Did the housekeepers have what they needed to do their best work? Merkt decided to tackle the question head on. At first, he observed Lead Environmental Services Aide, Denise Wolfe, a 30-year veteran at St. Margaret's, as she performed her morning duties. Within days, Merkt showed up in his scrubs to work side by side with Wolfe, to experience, first hand, some of the difficulties and begin to solve problems alongside her.

"It made me nervous at first," said Wolfe, "to have people watching me. Usually people come to watch you because they're trying to find you doing something wrong. But I realized that they were there to find ways to help me, and they did help. So I let them watch now, no problem. It's kind

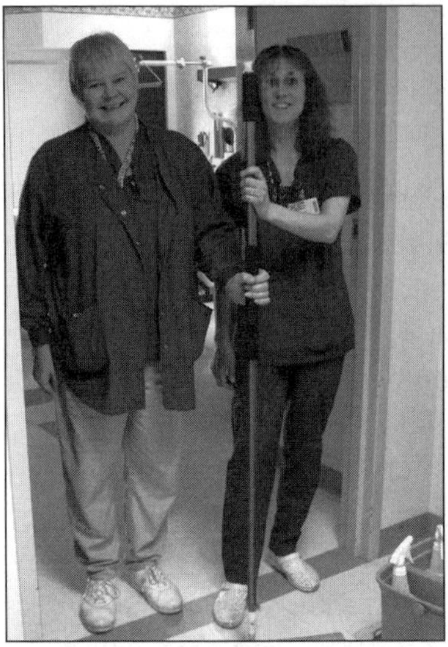

Figure 3-1. It's all about honoring the worker: 30-year veteran Denise Wolfe stands by Lisa Thomas.

of an honor that they care enough to show up to watch me and help." (See Figure 3-1.)

Heavy carts, heavy buckets

The housekeeping cart is laden with cleaning supplies and accompanied by a wheeled, stainless steel bucket filled with cleaning solution, and a dense mop head. The bucket assembly and wet string-mop weigh over 40 pounds (Figure 3-2, Table 3-1). Simply traveling to the room means that the housekeeper must push the heavy cart with one hand, and pull the heavy bucket assembly with the other. When the bucket water must be changed, at the completion of every third room, the aide must roll the bucket down the hall to the utility sink, lift it, pour it out, and refill it.

Table 3-1. Bucket Assembly Weights.

Bucket Assembly Weights	
Filled Bucket	27.5 lbs.
Wet Mop	4.4 lbs.
Wringer	9.1 lbs.
Total Assembly Weight	41 lbs.

Watching the housekeeping routine for an hour clarified the improvement potential. The possibility for worker injury was just too high as Denise's occasional backaches testified.

"Denise has been a leader on our housekeeping staff for 30 years. You can't find people like her. Every person on our housekeeping staff is irreplaceable. We needed to make their work easier," said Merkt. "I started researching other cleaning options."

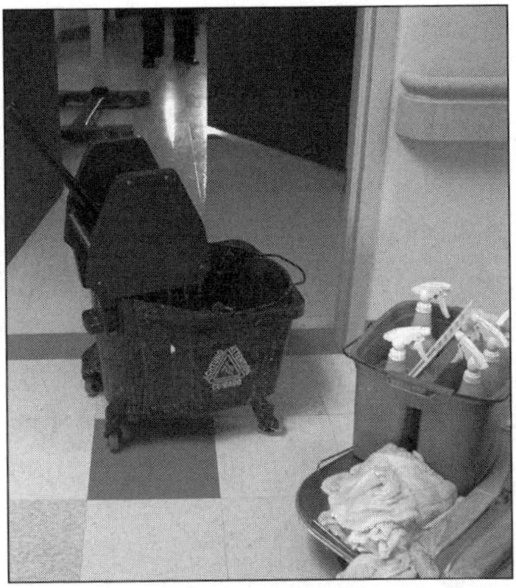

Figure 3-2. It was time to kick the bucket! With a total weight of 41 pounds, no wonder the bucket assembly has proven physically burdensome for workers.

A better mop

Merkt found an industrial model mop similar to the lightweight mops with microfiber heads so popular in households. The mop handle holds cleaning solution, dispensed by a trigger on the handle (Figure 3-3). Filled and ready for action, the mop weighs just over two pounds.

It took a little getting used to. At first, Wolfe was not enamored of the swiveling head. It seemed awkward. But within a few days, the benefits became more and more apparent. Ordinarily, the aide dry-mops the floor to remove debris, then wet-mops to disinfect. The new mop allows the aides to perform both operations in one pass. The new, wider mop head is more effective at removing dirt and debris. Because the mop head can be changed frequently, and because the cleaning solution is always clean, the floors in patient rooms are cleaner.

In an unexpected windfall, Merkt discovered a significant cost saving: The microfiber mop heads are far easier and less expensive to launder. The annual savings run into the thousands of dollars.

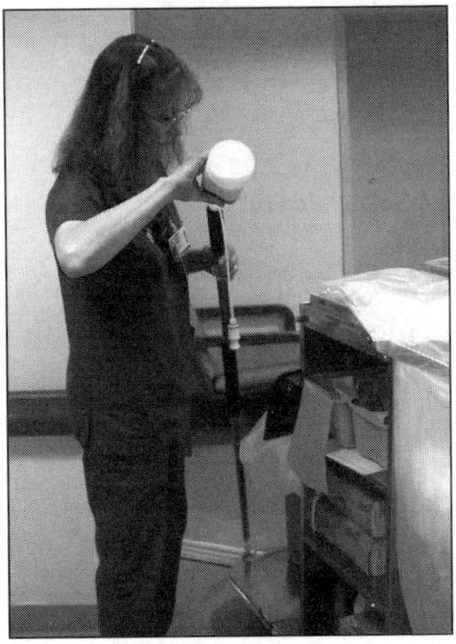

Figure 3-3. Environmental Services Aide, Lisa Thomas, fills the mop handle with cleaning solution. Filled and ready to go, the mop weighs just 2.3 lb (Bonus: solution is always clean; dry and wet mopping can be done in one operation. Microfiber mop heads are much less expensive to launder.)

A little safer, a little cleaner

Wolfe's subsequent observations revealed other opportunities to experiment with processes. While she wiped the surfaces of the room according to a set guideline, she had to make numerous trips back to the cleaning cart in the hallway to wring or change her cleaning cloth. To simplify the procedure, she prepared Ziploc bags with the necessary number of cleaning cloths for one room, premoistened with cleaning solution. When she enters a room, she brings a bag full of clean cloths, and an empty bag for the "dirties." After working out some initial bugs in the system, Wolfe now finds the cleaning routine shorter and more thorough, and the disruption to patients minimized.

"When a system is working well, the work is less hard," says Thompson. "When the right thing is easy to do, everybody wins."

The new mops and cleaning cloth procedures are catching on with the other housekeepers. Initial reluctance is being overcome as the convenience and time savings becomes apparent.

Less touching

Merkt and his staff realize that infection is most often transmitted on the hands of the healthcare worker. During observations, housekeeping staff were among the most likely to adhere scrupulously to hand hygiene requirements.

Still, Merkt looks for ways to reduce the possibility of transmission. "Every time you can eliminate the need for people to touch things, you reduce opportunities to transmit infection," said Merkt.

His department installed proximity-sensing towel dispensers that produce a clean paper towel after hand washing, with just the wave of a hand (Figure 3-4).

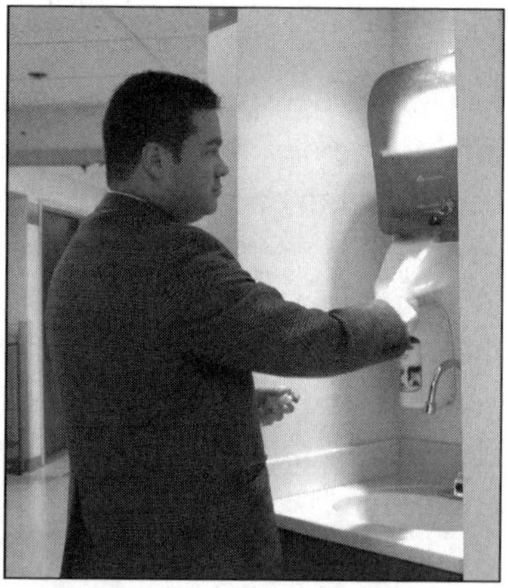

Figure 3-4. With a wave of the hand, new proximity-sensing towel dispensers produce a clean paper towel after handwashing, as Environmental Services Director, John Merkt demonstrates.

Looking for more such opportunities, Merkt recently had sensor-activated lights installed in supply rooms, so staff members never have to touch a light switch.

"Our housekeeping staff is so professional," says Merkt, "that they welcome improvements. Not only are they safer from injury, but patients are safer every time we figure out how to make a room a little cleaner."

Preparation for a larger response

Members of the Environmental Services department at UPMC St. Margaret had become accustomed to rapid-cycle improvements and refinements to their own work. Using Perfecting Patient Care techniques as part of everyday work prepared them to respond quickly to an uptick in the hospital's rate of clostridium difficile (*C. difficile*) infections. These infections are on the rise nationally. *C. difficile* is a bacterium that causes inflammation of the colon and diarrhea in patients, usually after they've been on antibiotics. Like MRSA, *C. difficile* is one of the more common hospital-acquired infections, although a virulent community-acquired strain is becoming prevalent as well.

In mid 2006, the hospital noted an increase in *C. difficile* cases, and responded by assembling an interdisciplinary taskforce that included the Infection Control Medical Director, clinical pharmacists, physicians, physician assistants, nurses, infection control practitioners, and of course, the Environmental Services Director, John Merkt.

Of course, infection control procedures were in effect, such as washing hands with soap and water (*C. difficile* is the one exception, a time when alcohol hand rub does not work as well as soap and water), wearing personal protective equipment, and testing and isolating patients at the first sign of the disease. But enhanced room cleaning became a significant component of controlling the problem.

Lead Environmental Services Aide Rita Adrian, Merkt, and Infection Control Practitioner, Susan DiNucci, RN, created a wallet card to remind housekeepers of the proper room-cleaning order. The taskforce selected a pilot unit, 6A, where many surgical patients reside, for a trial of all the *C. difficile* reduction techniques, including the new cleaning techniques.

Using guidelines published by the Centers for Disease Control and Prevention (CDC), Merkt worked with Adrian, and the infection control practitioners to standardize the way every room was cleaned. After a full cleaning, done the same way in the same order every time, the environmental services aide went over all "high touch" areas, like door handles, latches, bathroom fixtures, telephones, telemikes, and side rails, with a bleach-impregnated disposable wipe.

In addition to adopting an improved microfiber mop system, they change mop heads with each room. Staff also selected a special scrubber, microfiber mop that could clean the bathroom tile floor area thoroughly. Because microfiber is inexpensive to launder and sanitizes well, all cleaning cloths are now microfiber. Because the workers, themselves, suggested most of the changes, these enhancements were embraced. They had become accustomed to change as a way to improve their work.

Within three months, the rate of *C. difficile* on 6A began to decline (Figure 3-5). At the same time, the interdisciplinary team also looked at antibiotic use and selection as a means to reduce *C. difficile* infections. This may also have contributed to the reduction.

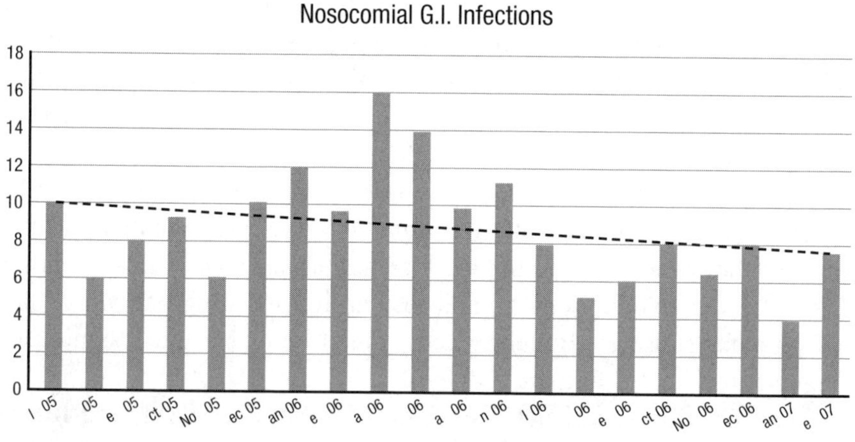

Figure 3-5. The rate of the hospital-acquired (nosocomial) gastrointestinal infection, *Clostridium difficile*, at UPMC St. Margaret declined once the interdisciplinary team standardized cleaning protocols, instituted CDC guidelines, and examined the use of antibiotics. Having been taught the basics of Perfecting Patient Care improvement techniques, the housekeepers made the changes quickly, suggesting most changes themselves.

The cleaning techniques rolled out gradually across the hospital. One by one, Adrian began going to the units, where she worked side by side with housekeepers for two full weeks to train them.

"We didn't do the roll-out all at once," explained Merkt. "We had to do it as quality would permit, so it took some time, but all the work is standardized now."

Adrian was nominated for an "Above and Beyond" award at the hospital for her work on this project. Soon the entire improvement cycle will start again, with videotaping of the cleaning process.

"It took awhile to standardize, but since July 2006, patient rooms in all units are being cleaned the same way," said Merkt. "If there's a problem, we know where to start looking and how to fix it."

• SECTION 2 •

PUTTING NURSES IN THE DRIVER'S SEAT

No one disputes this nation's nursing shortage. Nationally, nursing is one of the top professions undergoing attrition due to baby boomers' retirements. Fewer nurses are entering the profession at a time when more are needed than ever. In the Pittsburgh region, the turnover rate in nursing and allied professions hovers at about 5 percent—about the national average.

While policy makers everywhere scramble to find ways to retain and attract nurses, PRHI's parent Jewish Healthcare Foundation and the Robert Wood Johnson Foundation (RWJF) teamed up to try a regional experiment. In the resulting program, entitled Nurse Navigators, nine nurses would be trained and mentored using the principles of Perfecting Patient Care. The employers for the Nurse Navigators were given a small stipend to pay for the training time. For one year, these nurses would pursue an aspect of quality improvement in which they had a passionate interest.

The hypothesis was simple: When nurses are given the tools, scientific data-gathering skills, and permission to improve care at the bedside, they will be more satisfied in their work, and patients will receive measurably better care. Nurses win. Patients win.

The quality cornerstone of the Nurse Navigator program supports and complements the Magnet Program of the American Nurses Credentialing Center. Several area hospitals are pursuing Magnet status, part of which includes training nurses on how to collect data at the bedside to measure improvement. This is one of the most daunting aspects of the Magnet program, and also of Perfecting Patient Care.

"The thought of having to collect data at first seems to nurses as if we're making them do math calculations in the midst of giving care. But that's not it," said PRHI's Debra Thompson, MSN, RN, who mentored the Nurse Navigators. "The data can be very simple, but very relevant. Just knowing how many minutes something takes, or how many patients need a certain thing every day, can help point the way to improvement."

The next two case studies arose from the Nurse Navigator program, held throughout 2006. Thompson, the on-site coach and mentor, was involved with PRHI for over five years. She visited each of the nine sites periodically during the year, helping nurses understand how to collect data at the bedside. Other PRHI staff coaches included Mimi Falbo, MSN, RN, and Lexie Alton, RN.

Standardizing Nurses' Orders

"Reactive care isn't going to work any more," says Albert Minjock, MSN, RN, CCRN, FCCM, a nurse administration unit director at the University of Pittsburgh Medical Center (UPMC) Shadyside and Presbyterian Hospitals. "In the last 20 years, despite technological gains, overall patient outcomes have not improved."

Minjock's Nurse Navigator project was entitled, "Nurse-driven, goal-directed therapy," which is a way of saying it's time to let the nurses take charge of immediate bedside care. For many in the healthcare professions, letting nurses take charge is a revolutionary idea.

Minjock's approach gives nurses the wherewithal to research the sources of problems they encounter and fix them, one by one, according to the scientific method. Perfecting Patient Care training complemented his approach. The training taught methods of detailed, first-hand observation as a way of getting to the root of the problem at hand.

In the intensive care unit (ICU), where time is of the essence, a few minutes can mean the difference between recovery, permanent damage, and patient death. Research shows that the period of critical illness, when the most damage is done, usually lasts just an hour. But in a timed trial, Minjock's observations revealed that it takes an average of 33.8 minutes for a nurse to recognize a problem, page a physician, receive a return call, and start an intervention. This half hour does not account for "languish time," looking for supplies and information (Table 3-2). It adds up to this: Even under the best of circumstances, the patient is halfway to a potentially bad outcome before the nurse can act.

What if, in Minjock's words, the nurses had the keys to the car? Certain urgent therapies could be standardized, so when a critical care nurse recognizes a problem, he or she can start a standardized therapy protocol immediately. By the time the physician returns the call, the nurse has a much more complete picture of the problem to present, and has begun critical therapy much sooner.

Table 3-2. The Critical Hour.

The Critical Hour	
Research shows that the period of critical illness, when most damage is done, usually lasts just 1 hour. *Problem:* From the moment of recognition to the start of intervention took over half of that critical hour. (*N*=175)	
Problem recognition until paged	3.7 minutes
Page till call is returned	17.8 minutes
Call return to intervention	12.3 minutes
Average time from recognition to intervention	**33.8 minutes**

"It's real-time problem solving at the point of care," said Minjock. Echoing Dr. Shannon's findings (Chapter 2, Section 2), Minjock discovered, "Perfecting Patient Care isn't just about having the right supplies or saving steps, although those are very important things. My big finding is that, when it's applied clinically, it works."

Creating flow charts and standardized protocols for commonly confronted conditions required teamwork, education, supplies, and some startup capital. In return, not only do patients receive urgent care sooner, but, in line with additional research, certain other practices are being stopped.

"There is no evidence base for some of the things we do, like repeat CT scans after strokes, daily chest x-rays in intubated patients, or daily labs in patients without diagnosed metabolic disorders," said Minjock. "So we stopped."

Data on the first 100 patients following implementation of nurse-driven, goal-directed therapy, were better than expected. The average ICU stay declined by just over two days. Ventilator usage decreased by between 12 to 26 hours. Length of stay in the ICU was reduced by over three days. In all, over 292 ICU days were saved, and over $1.4 million in ICU bed costs alone (Table 3-3).

"Nurses working on this project are being recruited to speak at physicians' grand rounds across the community," said Minjock. "It's a gratifying acknowledgement that patient care starts at the bedside."

Table 3-3. Initial Results After Standardizing Nursing Protocol.

Initial Results After Standardizing Nursing Protocol	
(*N*=100; study period, Nov. 2005—Nov. 2006)	
Average ICU reduction in stay	2.2 days
Decrease in ventilator usage	12–26 hours
Average reduction in ICU length of stay based on scoring against control group	–3.17 days
Overall savings: ICU days	297
Overall savings in ICU alone	$1.4 million

• SECTION 3 •

STOPPING THE REVOLVING DOOR ON NURSING TURNOVER

Ordinarily, nursing turnover in the UPMC system is lower than the national average—3 percent instead of 5 percent. Distressing data emerged, however, from the abdominal transplant unit during 2004 and 2005: Nursing turnover had risen to a whopping 12 percent.

Christopher Saunders, BSN, RN, wanted to know why, and how to stop the exodus. This inquiry formed the basis of his 2006 Nurse Navigator project to stop the revolving door on nurse turnover.

"The loss of intellectual capital is the worst part," said Saunders. "But the financial costs were staggering, too." Saunders determined that it costs the institution about $40,000 for orientation of a new nurse on the transplant unit, and that the loss of nurses had cost about $880,000 over 2004–2005.

Saunders' deliberate observations on the unit identified bottlenecks in the system and other forms of waste. The effort fanned out in many directions. For example, professional practice councils and unit-based committees gave nurses a voice in managing patient care. The project piloted partnerships between nurse and aide, better coordinated discharge planning, divided the acutely ill patients more evenly, and modified the patient-to-nurse ratio. Health unit coordinators performed a "Clean Sweep" and reorganization of paper flow at the unit station. To reduce the time nurses spent running from patient to patient in rooms on each end of the unit, they were assigned patients in the same proximity (Figure 3-6a & b). Each patient room now has its own message board, and its own supply cart, linens, and hampers, which are always stocked.

These process improvements on their own began to create a more orderly work environment. But it was in "drilling down" into the details of work that the most dramatic and fastest progress was made.

For example, Saunders discovered that the abdominal transplant unit was not using Eclypsis, an electronic medical record in use at UPMC intensive care units for over a decade. The reason? Current staff needed training in its use. Training occurred, and then a few nurses piloted Eclypsis in a four-bed area. Almost immediately, the nurses discovered they

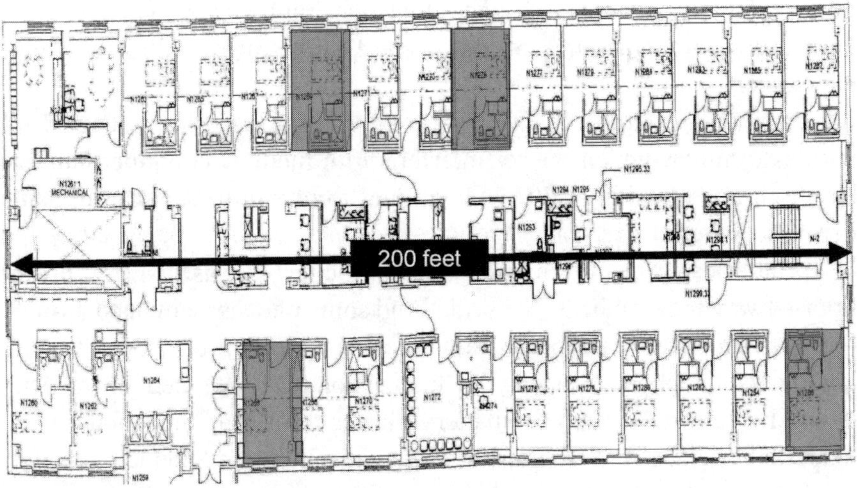

Figure 3-6a. Initial observation revealed nurses' patients geograpically dispersed, necessitating a lot of running.

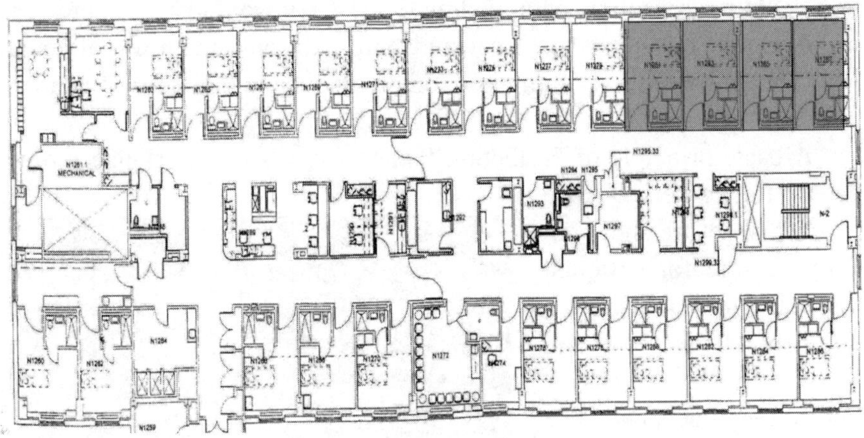

Figure 3-6b. Centralizing nurses' assignments, and making sure nobody has the most acutely ill patients, saves time for nurses and creates a better work environment.

saved time and shared better information with the physicians over the network. The nurses embraced Eclypsis, and its use quickly expanded from the four-bed pilot to the full 12-bed capacity.

Said Saunders, "One nurse estimated that using the Eclypsis system was saving her an hour a day—an hour she was able to apply to some other aspect of patient care. In essence, that one improvement gave an extra hour a day to every nurse on the floor. That result definitely improves patient care."

Another question arose: Why weren't the nurses using Spectra Link wireless phones, which do not interfere with medical equipment? Using the discipline of asking "Why?" five times to reveal the root cause, Saunders discovered the reason.

"Batteries were missing and only one charger was working on the floor—two wings, 54 beds," he said. "And some phones were just missing."

The administration replaced equipment and the staff developed a phone log to track the phones, posting the numbers on the assignment board. They devised a failsafe system for battery charging. "Communication among nurses, physicians, and lab improved dramatically," said Saunders.

Saunders had learned a "distress call" technique that allowed a unit that was overwhelmed with work to post a red flag that would suspend additional admissions for an hour. However, Saunders knew the transplant unit could never stop receiving admissions. They would have to intercept problems one by one, as they occurred, before the entire unit was affected.

"One nurse has to become 'red' before the whole unit does," Saunders reasoned.

A basic principle of Perfecting Patient Care is that workplaces must be safe for workers to voice problems before they can truly be safe for patients. What if individual nurses could hoist their own red flags when they were feeling overwhelmed, and have other nurses and even managers show up to assist them? Using children's toy flags, nurses began putting out green, yellow, and red flags at their locations to denote the status of their workload (Figure 3-7).

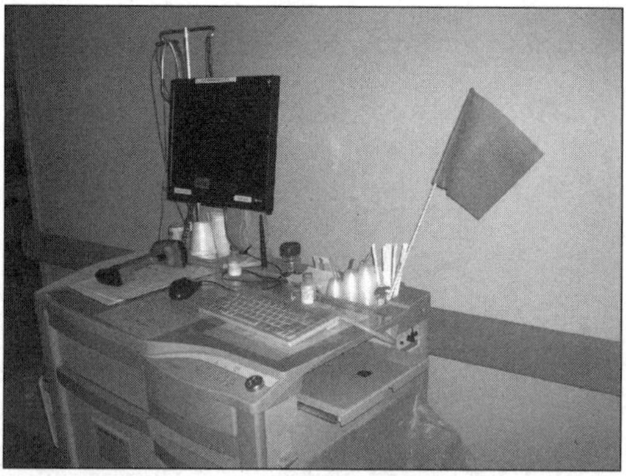

Figure 3-7. Hoisting the flag. This flag is green, indicating a nurse is within his or her working comfort zone. Nurses who raise yellow or red flags need help; those "in the green" quickly come to help.

Soon, nurses in the green would look for others posting yellow or red, and would go help out immediately. Nurses thrived on the ability to call out problem times with impunity, and count on help to arrive immediately. Teamwork, collegiality, and mutual support thrived in this atmosphere. The color-coding system quickly and spontaneously spread to other units.

Taken together, the measures made a large collective difference in work flow. But did it make enough difference to the nurses to make them want to stay?

Since the inception of Saunders' Nurse Navigator Program in January 2006, turnover on the abdominal transplant unit has been zero (Table 3-4).

Table 3-4. RN Turnover Rates on Abdominal Transplant Unit.

RN Turnover Rates on Abdominal Transplant Unit	
Year	**Number of RN resignations**
2003	3
2004	12 (12 percent)
2005 (Jan-Sept)	10
Jan 2006 (PPC innovations begun) to Dec 2006	0

CHAPTER 4

Making Handoffs Safer

CASE STUDIES

- **Section 1. Eliminating tangled lines leads to other improvements.** The symptom: tangled intravenous (IV) lines following cardiac surgery. Solving the problem meant reviewing every handoff from admission through discharge.
- **Section 2. Safer shift change.** High-tech and low-tech ways of imparting more complete information about each patient to the next shift more quickly.
- **Section 3. Eliminating patient falls.** Better handoffs reduce falls.

A 2005 study attributes faulty communication to nearly 70 percent of hospital mishaps. Other studies have shown that at least half of all such communication breakdowns happen during the change of shift.[1]

Peter Angood, MD, vice president and chief patient safety officer for the Joint Commission's International Center for Patient Safety said, "JCAHO (Joint Commission on Accreditation of Healthcare Organizations) has gathered a decade's worth of data related to sentinel event activity—and a common theme that's always at the top is the issue of communication. And one of the most important areas is handoff. It's a high-risk period, and there is a tendency to undercommunicate."[2]

High-stakes handoffs occur regularly in other industries: air traffic control to ground control; industrial equipment changeovers; and racecar pit crews. Applying techniques from industry can improve the scope and speed of communications. It requires many of the techniques taught in Toyota-based systems like Perfecting Patient Care.

---

1. Gautam Naik, "A Hospital Races To Learn Lessons of Ferrari Pit Stop," *Wall Street Journal*, page A1, (November 14, 2006).
2. "JCAHO to look closely at patient handoffs: communication lapses will be key focus," *HealthCare Benchmarks and Quality Improvement* (Dec, 2005).

• SECTION 1 •

ELIMINATING TANGLED LINES LEADS TO OTHER IMPROVEMENTS

When a patient is admitted to a hospital for coronary artery bypass graft (CABG) surgery, he or she begins a multistop tour through the hospital system. Some hospital designers have wondered why the patient—the person in need of care—doesn't remain in one place while all services come to him or her. Instead, the patient "travels" from the medical unit to the presurgery area to surgery to the intensive care unit (ICU) to the intermediate step-down unit and finally, home.

During any one of these handoffs between units, confused information and inconsistent processes can place the patient at increased risk of error. In his Physician Champion program, Michael H. Culig, MD, a cardiothoracic surgeon who has been engaged with the work of PRHI for nearly a decade, wanted to apply Perfecting Patient Care methods to ensure smoother transfers of postsurgical patients to the ICU, thus minimizing the time they are under sedation or on ventilation, while improving outcomes and reducing complications. This work became the basis of his 2006–2007 Physician Champion grant.

The technique always begins with the question, *Why can't we?* This question challenges participants to work toward an ideal condition or state, removing the barriers to improvement. In the case of postsurgical care for cardiac patients, the questions became, *Why can't we . . .*

- Perfect communication between all nursing units and the operating room (OR), ensuring that every patient arrives at the OR on time, in perfect condition, with the preoperative antibiotic administered?
- Ensure every patient has a perfect transfer to intensive care unit (ICU)?
- Effect perfect patient transfers from ICU to the intermediate step-down unit?
- Follow up with patients to confirm whether or not each person had experienced a perfect discharge?

In one example, on transfer from surgery to the ICU, patients often arrive with tangled intravenous (IV) lines. The question was, "*Why can't we* ensure that every patient arrives in the ICU with perfect lines?" Answering the question and untangling the lines involved working with everyone in the work pathway—from surgery, transport, and ICU—to find a way to solve the problem.

Step 1: First pass at identifying problem, 2002–2003

Untangling the lines took over 25 minutes of RN time—a waste and a nuisance. But far worse, tangled IV lines represented a potential hazard for the patient (Figure 4-1). A group of workers teamed up to solve the problem. The ICU director, nurses, nurse anesthetists, and support generalists convened to discuss ways to make transfer from the OR to the ICU flawless.

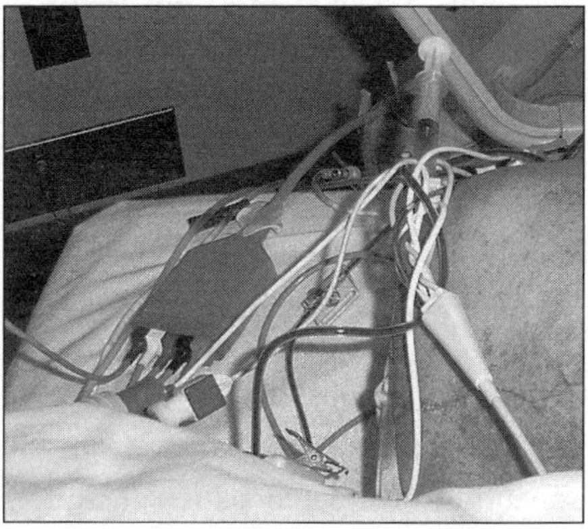

Figure 4-1. Step 1: Assess the current condition. Problem: patient arrives in ICU with tangled IV lines. RNs must spend 25 minutes to untangle them. The confusion poses risk for patients.

Step 2: Define the ideal condition

Using a mannequin, (Figure 4-2) the nurses collaborated to show the other team members their *ideal condition* in which patients should arrive at the ICU. They showed every detail, including placement of incoming and outgoing lines and IV bags.

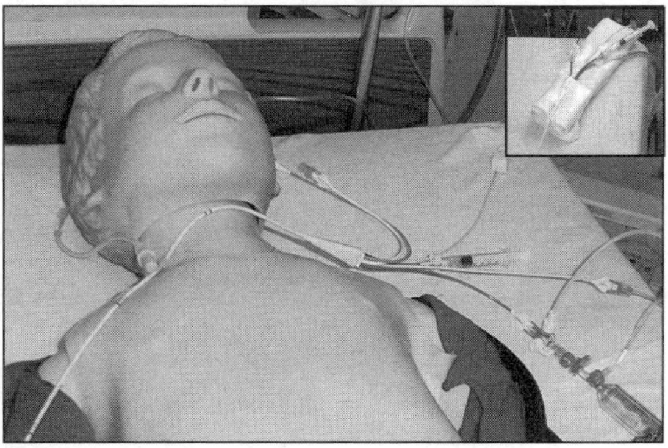

Figure 4-2. Step 2: Create a picture of the ideal situation. In this case, the team used a mannequin and a "Swan Pillow." The work continues on process improvement with every transfer.

Step 3: Find the root cause—the Five Whys

Why couldn't the ideal condition be met? On its journey to the root cause of the problem, the team asked, "Why?" five times. Repeating this question led them to discover: In the OR, the IV bags are held on two poles. During transfer, the bags are all loaded onto one. The tangle begins. During transfer from the OR to the ICU, the oxygen bottle is placed at the foot of the bed, under the patient's feet. This leaves only one place for the heart monitor: by the patient's shoulder, on top of the IV lines, with the screen facing away from the person transporting the patient (Figure 4-3).

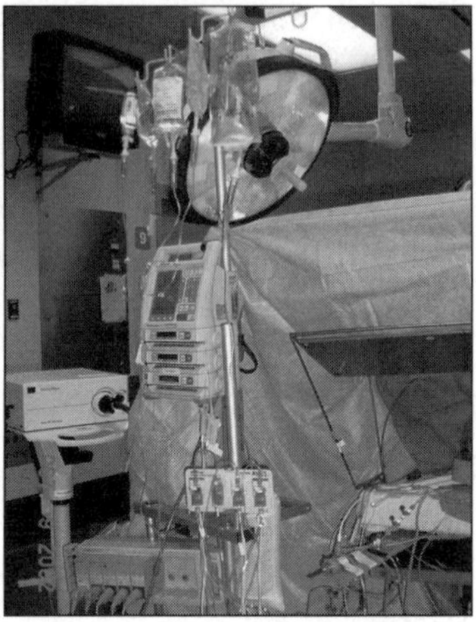

Figure 4-3. Step 3: Determine the root cause (5 Whys). Two IV poles hold separate banks of IVs in the OR. When all bags are placed on just one IV pole for transport, the tangle begins.

Step 4: Design countermeasures

The IV bags needed to be kept separated during transport—in left and right banks, just as in the OR. A nurse suggested using the bed's IV pole to transfer one bank of IV bags, and a wheeled IV pole for the other.

The heart monitor needed to be held off the bed, off the patient, and off the IV lines during transport. A nurse anesthetist suggested using the portable table designed for the end of the bed. An added benefit: the screen now faces the transporter (Figure 4-4).

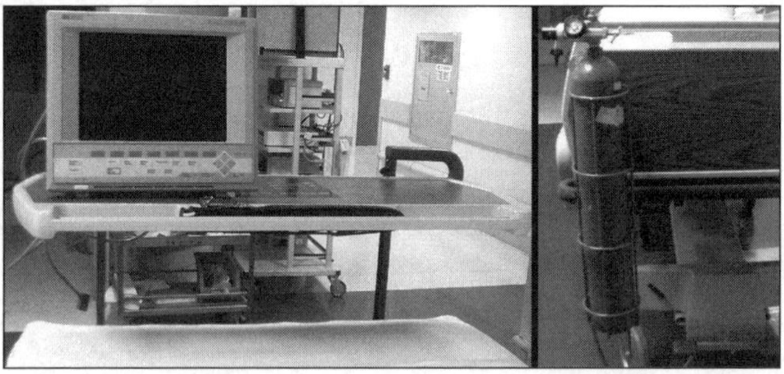

Figure 4-4. Step 4: Countermeasures. The heart monitor now rests on a table mounted to the foot of the bed—off the IV lines and visible to the person transporting the patient. The oxygen bottle now rests in a bed-mounted basket designed for that purpose.

The technician discovered a previously unused bed accessory made to hold the oxygen bottle and installed it on the beds used to transport CABG patients.

Solving one problem to its root cause allowed a team to address a host of issues, resulting in safer transfer of patients following heart surgery, and incidentally, saving valuable time of healthcare workers.

Refine and refresh

Now, keeping lines untangled has become part of a surgical checklist. IV lines are organized toward the end of the operation and arranged so that when the patient arrives in the ICU, confusion, effort, and time are minimized. Initially, the ICU nurses were gratified, and all on the team came to recognize the importance of the work. Nurse time spent fixing the IV lines on transfer went from 25 minutes to less than five, reducing the "hassle factor" for the nurses, but more important, making it much safer for patients.

"When things go wrong, confusion over the lines can be one of those things in a cascade of events that leads to catastrophe," says Dr. Culig. "Having quick, easy access to the correct line—that single improvement—can keep the cascade from unfolding and avert a bigger problem. When we systematically eliminate each part of a complex problem, we create a much safer environment for patients."

The problem of tangled lines was initially tackled in 2003. However, maintaining the progress proved difficult. Employee turnover diluted the collective understanding of the problem. In 2006, Dr. Culig received a grant from the Jewish Healthcare Foundation to continue his work applying these Toyota-based techniques to handoffs. He aims to create, "A culture in the OR and each nursing unit where enough individuals understand the power of work redesign that they will develop their own responses, so they have ownership, and it won't be something imposed from outside."

Work continues on the crucial transfer from the OR to the ICU. One experiment involved specifying physician assistants (PAs) as transfer experts who oversee every aspect of a patient's transfer. Initial results with this approach look promising. Work continues on ways to trigger PA involvement.

Other factors can create a less-than-perfect transfer. The group has discovered that the transfer of a patient to the intermediate step-down unit comes with a potential for medication error. Changes made in the regimen while the patient is readied in the ICU for transfer that can create problems in the intermediate step-down unit. Again applying principles of Perfecting Patient Care, and increasing communication between the ICU and step-down unit continue to improve worker satisfaction, along with patient safety.

Dr. Culig believed that confusion at discharge led some patients to be readmitted or have less-than-perfect outcomes. He hired a nurse to call patients the day after they went home to perform a medication reconciliation with the patient, comparing what had been ordered in the hospital to what the patient was taking.

"There was a lot of confusion," said Dr. Culig. "In many cases, medications had not been ordered or were not being taken properly."

Patients are now seen in their homes one to two weeks after discharge. These visits have helped reconcile additional medication problems and confusion. Some incipient infections have been caught early, preventing several patients from having to be readmitted.

While the concept may be simple, work redesign is difficult. Dr. Culig believes it's worth the effort. "There's no doubt about it: When handoffs are smoother, patients have better outcomes."

• SECTION 2 •

SAFER SHIFT CHANGE

It's coming up on 3 PM and, as usual, the unit has been very busy today. But each nurse simply must take the time to report on what's gone on with each patient, so the nurse assuming the next shift will be informed. Often, what's reported are the subtle things—things that may not even make it into the patient's chart. And it's important to impart the information as close as possible to the actual shift change, when the information is the most up to date.

The problem is that, just because the nurses need about a half hour to convey this information to one another, doesn't mean that the patients stop having needs during that time. In fact, one hospital tracked a distinct spike in the number of patient falls during the period surrounding shift change.

And what was the typical shift change like for nurses? At UPMC Shadyside and the VA Pittsburgh Healthcare System (VAPHS), nurses relied on tape-recorded updates about individual patients—reports that everyone hoped would be sufficient.

"Everybody hurried and scrambled," said Susan Christie Martin, RN, at UPMC Shadyside. "Staff looked for recorders, what their assignment was. Tape recorders helped, but sometimes you couldn't find one, or the battery was dead, or the cord was missing. You could never find your place if you rewound."

"Taped information wasn't standardized," said Ellesha McCray, MSN., RN, of the VAPHS. "Nurses gave what they thought were the most salient points, but sometimes important bits of information were skipped."

Clearly, the system of conveying information at shift change presented opportunities to improve employee satisfaction and patient safety. UPMC Shadyside and the VAPHS, two Pittsburgh-area hospitals in different systems, tackled and streamlined shift change: UPMC using an advanced voicemail system; VAPHS using an all-encompassing form that has since become computerized.

Both hospitals were aiming toward what in a Toyota-based system is called the "ideal condition": a perfect shift change, where *all* and *only* the required information gets passed to the right people, at the right time, in a standardized way that supports best-practice care. Although their methods varied, both hospitals reported measurable time savings and improvement in the quality of information exchanged at shift change.

UPMC SHADYSIDE

Nurses report their satisfaction with the Voicecare system, a telephonic answer to the use of tape recorders. UPMC Shadyside piloted the system on two units, and based on high satisfaction, expanded its use. The system offers several advantages: The nurse can report on patients, one by one, as soon as they have been seen. Using a desktop or pocket phone in a secure, confidential area, the nurse signs in with a firewall-protected user code and dictates the report for that shift into that patient's secure mailbox.

Information is standardized: For example, the system prompts the user to enter the patient's history, which is then saved. (In the days of tape recorders, patient histories had to be rerecorded at the end of every shift.) The second prompt is for what is happening with the patient today. In the third area, nurses can enter addenda regarding the myriad other things that the next nurse may find important or useful. These addenda can be made at any time, any time the nurse visits the patient.

Currently, nurses use Voicecare for shift report, but the system is now being rolled out for use as patients come to and from procedural labs, and from pre-op to post-op. It's catching on in other areas, too. An authorized physician in an outlying office can call and get a report on a hospitalized patient, and can dictate a report into the phone to let nurses know about that patient. Emergency Department physicians call reports into patients' Voicecare phones when a patient is transferred to the floor to convey details of the patient's initial encounter. Certain long-term care facilities to which UPMC Shadyside patients most often transfer also receive passwords so that they can hear the Voicecare hospitalization reports when the patient arrives from the hospital. Voicecare reports can be recalled for up to 20 hours after the patient is discharged.

Just who may do the calling into the Voicecare system? The hospital has experimented with allowing family members to dial into the system to hear the Voicecare reports. While many families appreciate access to this information, it does not reduce the family's need to talk with a member of the healthcare team.

Results

As Figure 4-5 shows, ultimately the two units reported a net decrease of 2.5 minutes per report. The extrapolated time savings over one year is estimated at 10,768 hours per year.

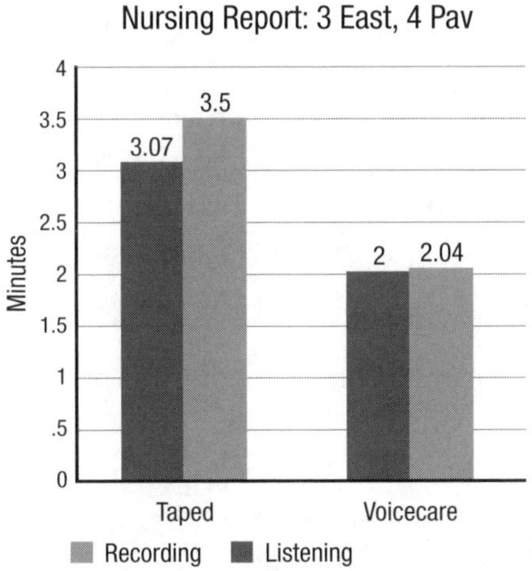

Figure 4-5. Decreased Reporting Time and Increased Accuracy of Information with Voicecare System.

VETERANS ADMINISTRATION PITTSBURGH HEALTHCARE SYSTEM

From a decidedly low-tech start, the VAPHS's shift-change procedure has proven a revelation for caregivers and a benefit for patients. Conveying information during a typical shift change on the 4 West pilot unit at the VAPHS, as at most other hospitals, took between 45 and 60 minutes.

The first step toward streamlining the process involved a stopgap measure that immediately cut the required time. VAPHS divided the entire unit's tape-recorded reports into two halves, so nurses only needed to listen to the half pertaining to their patients. Yet, the team discovered that even after listening to 30 or 45 minutes of information, the nurses still spent a lot of time seeking information on the computer, in the charts and in the Kardex system. Could the team both combine and streamline the information from all sources?

The group decided to apply the quick changeover methods used routinely in industry. This process concentrates on getting the right information in the right order to the right people at the right time. After examining the current condition, the group asked a few penetrating questions:

- Is all of this work necessary for the changeover? (For example, must nurses listen to reports on patients for whom they will not be caring?)
- What information do nurses actually need?
- Must all the information be exchanged in the shift report, or at the time of need in a different way? Two categories of necessary information are: general assessment (vitals, history) and diagnosis-specific (best-practice care for each condition).

In keeping with the Perfecting Patient Care principle of standardized work, nurses decided to create a form that would convey necessary information in the same order every time. Doing so creates a logical way to give and receive information, and makes missing information more obvious. This form evolved into a laminated card for each patient and served as a checklist for care.

Despite computerization, nurses still relied on the Kardex system for certain information. They reconfigured the Kardex form in an efficient layout with all, and only, pertinent information. (This revised Kardex form spread quickly to other units. It was not "pushed" or recommended by managers, but was quickly assumed by rank-and-file nurses who demanded the improvement.)

Regarding diagnosis-specific information, nurses determined that most patients on their floor suffered from about 36 common diagnoses. In teams of two, the nurses volunteered to review all information on best practices and create checklists for each condition. Over time, the nurses created comprehensive checklists for all 36 conditions.

"Pilots use checklists for the most common, everyday procedures to ensure safety. With complex medical care, nobody can remember every report item for every condition—nor should they," says Peter Perreiah, a PRHI Director who worked on the MRSA and other improvement projects in the unit for four years.

"Creating these checklists helps ensure that every patient receives best-practice care," says Ellesha McCray, RN, 4 West Team Leader. "Furthermore, the system greatly reduces the time required to convey information at shift change, which leaves more time for things like direct patient care and 100 percent hand hygiene."

A computerized version of the RN shift report uses pop-up menus to efficiently capture patient reports and support shift changeovers.

Results

The nurses on 4 West have reduced the briefing time at shift change from one hour to 15 minutes. Standardizing the briefings also improved their quality. The information is more complete and far more comprehensive, reducing time seeking subsequent and missing information. The VAPHS estimates annual time savings for the nurses on 4 West at about the equivalent of three full-time employees.

Patients benefit when nurses devote more time to them and less time seeking information. They also benefit when practitioners use a checklist that virtually guarantees best-practice care.

• SECTION 3 •

ELIMINATING PATIENT FALLS

Data from regional hospitals indicate that the number of patient falls, while small, represents a huge toll on patients and caregivers alike. Some hospitals track only falls that cause injury. Many more now track falls or near falls, in the hope that tracking "near-miss" data can help prevent injuries. One hospital discovered a spike in patient falls at shift change, and used that information to streamline the process, realizing that patients' needs—like the need for a bathroom break—do not stop for a shift change.

Led by a nurse and the CEO, one largely rural hospital, the 103-year-old, 225-bed Monongahela Valley Hospital, decided that the only acceptable goal for patient falls was zero.

MONONGAHELA VALLEY SYSTEMATICALLY REDUCES FALLS

Lynda Nester, MSN, RN, still remembers when her great-grandmother fell, broke her hip, and began an inexorable decline that led to her death some years later. Preventing falls is a passion with Nester, because even today, 25 percent of patients with hip fractures die within a year and only 25 percent fully recover.

Fortunately, her commitment is shared by top leadership at Monongahela Valley Hospital, where CEO Louis J. Panza, Jr., recently declared "zero falls" a hospital-wide goal. Enlisting everyone along the pathway of work, from the CEO to the vendors of slippers and beds, is Nester's idea of teamwork, and formed the basis of her effort, incorporating Perfecting Patient Care to prevent falls.

This fall-reduction program was aided by Nester's Nurse Navigator grant from the Jewish Healthcare Foundation of Pittsburgh, PRHI's parent organization. That program gave her training, on-site coaching, and help with data collection.

Although falls are costly, that was not the reason Nester decided to try to eliminate them. She knew that half of the patients at Monongahela Valley Hospital are at risk of falling, 25 percent at very high risk. The memories of her grandmother's decline increased her commitment to increase safety for these patients.

In Chapter 1, Steve Lares was not the only person injured by his fall out of a wheelchair. His nurse, Michelle, was emotionally upset by the event as well.

"Whether they result in injury or not, falls traumatize patients and they traumatize healthcare workers, too," said Nester. Nurses are devastated when harm comes to a patient. Evidence suggests that such events lead many nurses to leave the profession.

Using principles of Perfecting Patient Care, Nester and her team first described their "ideal condition" as "zero falls," and then began to observe vulnerable patients and nurses during critical times, including shift change. Their observations revealed that not every patient who needed a low bed had one. They found that patients did not feel free to stop an obviously busy nurse to ask for help shifting positions or getting out of bed to go to the bathroom. In an effort to spare a busy nurse, patients might try to get up by themselves.

High-tech and low-tech improvements

The team evaluated various high- and low-tech options for reducing risk, from color-coded patient wrist bands to low beds to alarms, to slipper socks with treads all the way around—the socks may slip, but the patient won't.

Vendors played a key role, along with nonclinical members of the care team. For example, when bed alarms habitually went off falsely, staff disarmed them. A visit from the vendor revealed the reason: The alarms were broken due to improper storage. The information was shared throughout the care team, and members of the maintenance department created hangers for the bed alarms, which stored them properly and made them easier to find and use. Bed alarms are again in routine use, and are always clean and available.

Low beds are of particular value, said Nester, and buying enough of them meant a significant investment on the part of the hospital. But instead of resistance in the purchasing department, she found kindred spirits who understood how terrible falls can be. The head of the department gave an impassioned plea for the low beds, and the number available is still increasing.

Standardizing communications

Above all, interdisciplinary communication propelled Nester's work. She created a check sheet to collect information on every fall or near-fall and summarized the results. Factors such as medication, cognition, and toileting came to the fore. (Figures 4-6; 4-7; 4-8.)

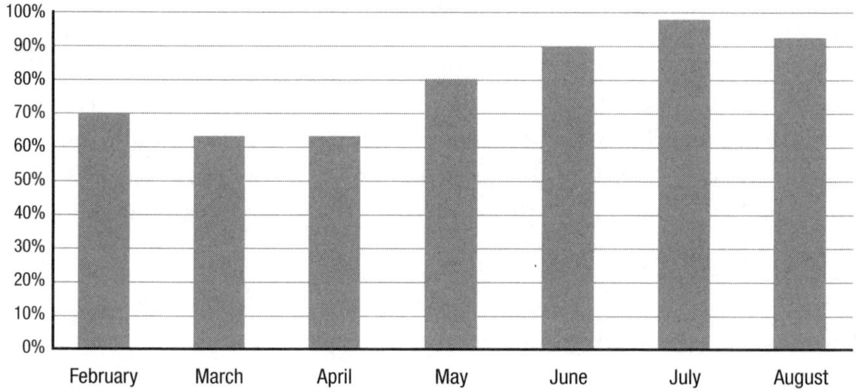

Figure 4-6. Medication as a Potential Contributing Factor in Patients Who Have Fallen.

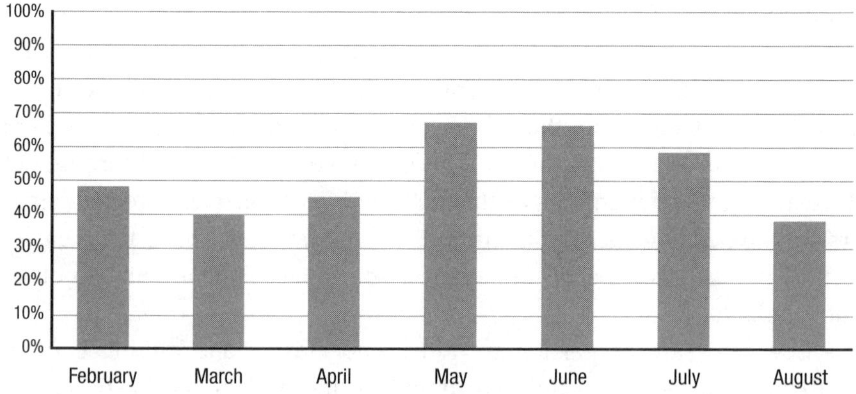

Figure 4-7. Toileting as a Contributing Factor in Patients Who Have Fallen.

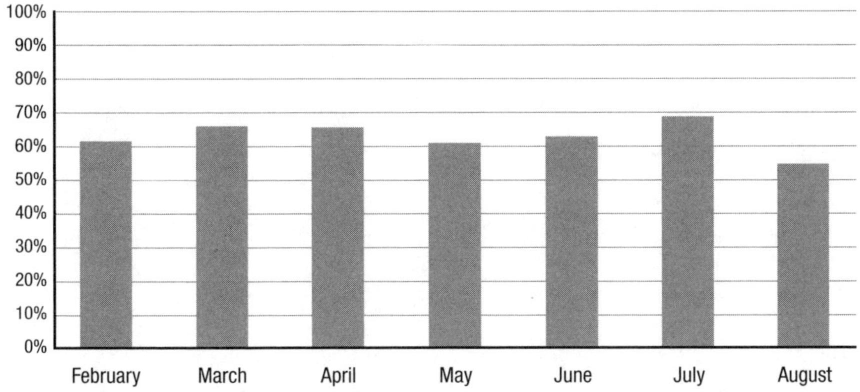

Figure 4-8. Presence of Delirium or Dementia, Psychiatric Diagnoses, or Drug and Alcohol Abuse in Patients who Fall.

The teams now have standardized the "5 Ps," a checklist for patients at risk of falling:

- Protect (with alarms and low beds)
- Pain (make sure it's managed)
- Potty (offer toileting)
- Position (ensure comfort)
- Provide (phone, water, education)

Before leaving a room, staff members are trained to stop and ask, "Is there anything else I can do for you?" and to assure patients that, "I have the time." With that kind of prompting, patients are more likely to ask for help, and less likely to try to get out of bed unassisted.

Standardized forms to identify patients' risks for falling are now discussed at every shift change. Nester realizes that's when many falls occur and is looking for ways to further streamline that process.

Results

Overall, falls at Monongahela Valley Hospital are down since Nester's intervention began. Six units have each celebrated a month or more with zero falls. One unit has gone five months without a fall.

CHAPTER 5

Reducing Medication Errors

CASE STUDIES

- **Section 1. Low-cost, low-tech pharmacy improvements.** Watch as two hospital pharmacies, UPMC South Side and LifeCare Hospitals of Pittsburgh, implement low-cost, low-tech quality improvements.
- **Section 2. Identifying every patient.** In a small community hospital where neighbors are the healthcare providers, not everyone feels the need to band every patient. It takes complete collaboration to change this culture.
- **Section 3. Secret of deploying high-tech machines: people first.** Getting medications to patients on time, 99 percent of the time, requires high-tech assistance—and sometimes the services of a plumber.

In Chapter 1, although Steve Lares suffered from a terminal illness, his death was caused by a medication error: the mismanagement of the anticoagulant, heparin. Anticoagulants are among the five most common medications in reported medication errors, according to a report cited by the Institute of Medicine.[1] That same report estimates that over 7,000 people die each year from medication errors in American hospitals. Over 770,000 people are injured or die each year from adverse drug reactions.[2] The cost of treating adverse drug reactions during hospitalization is estimated to range from $1.56 to $5.6 billion annually.[3]

Faced with the nearly overwhelming complexity of the healthcare system, the search for answers usually leans toward the high-tech panacea. Magical thinking leads to the latest computerized gadget, which usually seems like an appealing, one-size-fits-all, silver bullet.

---

1. Institute of Medicine (IOM), "To Err Is Human: Building a Safer Health System," (2000).

Sometimes, the breathtaking wizardry of advanced devices like computerized human body simulators, electronic medical record systems for patient records, and computerized physician order entry and barcode medication administration machinery to ensure medication safety is truly dazzling. It's estimated, for example, that computerized physician order entry can instantly reduce medication errors by over 90 percent—a quantum leap in anybody's language.

Yet two barriers remain: (1) small hospitals and small clinical practices cannot afford the advanced simulator, medical record and pharmaceutical technology; and (2) even with an immediate 90 percent reduction in medication error, that recalcitrant (although far more manageable) 10 percent remains.

In both cases—in all cases—it comes down to the people who do the work. The studies in this chapter (and the story on electronic medical records in Chapter 7) demonstrate that those who cannot afford the technology need not wait for it; and those who can afford it can still benefit from a disciplined, scientific approach to problem solving, inherent in systems like Perfecting Patient Care.

It begins and ends with the workers at the front line.

---

2. "Reducing and Preventing Adverse Drug Events To Decrease Hospital Costs." Research in Action, Issue 1. Publication Number 01-0020. Agency for Healthcare Research and Quality (AHRQ), Rockville, MD, (March 2001). http://www.ahrq.gov/qual/aderia/aderia.htm.

   See also: D. C. Classen et al., "Adverse drug events in hospitalized patients," *JAMA*277(4):301–306 (1997). D. J. Cullen et al., "Preventable adverse drug events in hospitalized patients: A comparative study of intensive care and general care units," *Crit Care Med* 25(8):1289–1297 (1997). D. J. Cullen et al., "The incident reporting system does not detect adverse drug events: A problem for quality improvement," *Journal on Quality Improvement* 21(10):541–548 (1995).
3. Ibid.

• SECTION 1 •

LOW-COST, LOW-TECH PHARMACY IMPROVEMENTS

Not every hospital can afford sophisticated pharmacy-tracking software. For smaller and community hospitals, advanced, but expensive, tools like computerized physician order entry or barcode medication administration may be years away. And while implementing these state-of-the-art programs can eliminate a whole host of problems, it can introduce others that can tax the problem-solving capabilities of an organization.

What low-cost, low-tech steps can a hospital take to begin to make medication administration safer? Two Pittsburgh-area hospitals have worked on some innovations using Perfecting Patient Care.

UPMC SOUTH SIDE PHARMACY: THE *UN*-BATCHING EXPERIMENT

"It's a matter of learning to look at work differently," says Kelley Wasicek, manager, pharmaceutical services, UPMC South Side, about Perfecting Patient Care as practiced in her unit. "Often it seems counterintuitive."

One of the most difficult and fundamentally different ways of looking at work is as a patient-focused "pull" system. Ordinarily, work is a series of tasks and demands placed upon workers by supervisors or others on up the chain of command. This system relies on "push"—push on the worker to produce, and push on the product to the customer, often regardless of whether the customer has a need for it.

An Example of Push

The pharmacy's method of unit dose batching aptly exemplifies a "push" system in action. The pharmacy filled, checked, and delivered all its intravenous (IV) orders up to 48 hours in advance and pushed them out. The problem was that, in that amount of time, patients were transferred or discharged and medication orders changed. The pharmacists had prepared medication to meet a need that, for one reason or another, no longer existed. Having numerous extra doses on the floor increased the chance for medication error. And in the end, a large percentage of the IV medication came right back to the pharmacy and required time-consuming restocking and crediting (Figure 5-1).

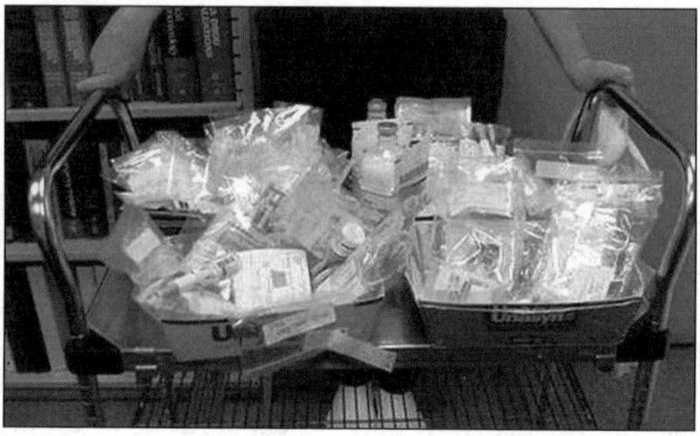

Figure 5-1. "We basically prepared all these IVs and took them out for a walk."—Kelley Wasicek, manager, pharmaceutical services, UPMC South Side.

"We basically prepared all these IVs and took them out for a walk," said Wasicek.

Moving Closer to the Ideal

Pharmacy staff members wanted to move closer to a system where their work would be "pulled" by their clients—the nurses (and ultimately, of course, the patients). Stated as the ideal condition, the patient "pulls" from the system what is needed. In the words of Toyota, such an ideal delivers what the patient needs in a way that is defect free, one by one, with no waste, immediately—in an environment that is physically, emotionally, and professionally safe. Preparing only what is needed, when it's needed reduces the potential for error and waste.

To move their system closer to the ideal, two years ago, the pharmacists examined their batching process and halved the advance time, from three days to 32 hours. Shortening the lead time resulted in a reduction in IV returns, to 25–39 percent. Still, pharmacy technicians wasted hours preparing and restocking IVs that were ultimately returned.

Wasicek and her team decided to experiment with shorter IV fill intervals. Acting on a main tenet of Perfecting Patient Care, "learning by doing," pharmacy staff began to experiment with the frequency and timing of filling and delivery. They shortened lead times to between 3 and 15 hours, depending on the scheduled administration time for a particular dose. Fewer than 17 percent of the IVs were then returned.

"The Pharmacy Department is not staffed 24 hours a day, so we have to do some preparation ahead of time," said Wasicek. "And while our system is still not ideal, we are providing meds much closer to 'just in time' and showing some good results."

The unbatching experiment is beginning to save time—five minutes here and five minutes there. It adds up. Based on previous observations, the batching experiment could save up to 89 minutes of pharmacist time and 13 hours of tech time per week.

"Now if we can figure out a way to 'batch' the saved time," says Wasicek, "that would seal our success."

Wasicek sees merit in this experiment because, "it's authentic work, not a contrived scenario. We try to engage everyone, including our customer, in the design of the work, then decide what's working and what's not."

Education and Training

Education is key for inquisitive pharmacists. Wasicek believes that the comfort level required for change can only be achieved through a thorough understanding of the underlying principles of work redesign. The pharmacy staff attended the Perfecting Patient Care University at PRHI, four full days of intensive instruction. Part of the instruction deals with the use of A-3s, the road maps that specify goals and methods (see sidebar).

On a practical level, each staff member has an opportunity to work as team leader, solving problems in the course of work.

What is an A-3?

It's no mystery. The term A-3 is the name given to 11″ by 17″ sheets of paper. A-3s are tools derived from the Toyota Production System (TPS). In Perfecting Patient Care, A-3s help map out problems as they exist, observe the current condition, define what the ideal situation would look like, hypothesize how to get from here to there, and build in tests.

Why use them?

A-3s provide a disciplined way of examining problems and creating solutions. In any Toyota-based methodology, every problem is mapped this way, usually by hand, and used as a springboard for specific actions and measurements of progress. PRHI has adopted the A-3 across all disciplines represented.

"We are learning the value of a good A-3," says Wasicek. "When you're not sure what to do, if you have a question or a problem, you can refer to the highly specified design on the A-3."

ELIMINATING ILLEGIBLE ORDERS AT LIFECARE

LifeCare Hospitals of Pittsburgh operates 196 beds and a medical staff of more than 200 physicians. LifeCare specializes in the treatment of medically complex patients who require extended hospitalization, typically for more than 25 days.

In May 2005, LifeCare's CEO threw down the gauntlet on illegible and incomplete pharmacy orders, setting the expectation that staff would work together to eliminate them. An improvement team of frontline doctors, nurses, and pharmacists began by addressing the basics: a clear order form. The existing form allowed for mostly free text. Hasty handwriting and incompleteness posed continual sources of confusion once the order reached the pharmacy.

The key to making the form easier lay in the "visual cue." With columns of information asking for drug-dose-route-frequency, missing information was immediately obvious. The first revision was introduced in mid-May, followed quickly by several revisions.

"It was the first time changes were made spontaneously, without seeking approval from a committee. It was also the first time that changes were made by the people doing the work rather than a group of leaders in a conference room," said pharmacy manager Darlene Schreiber. "The form dramatically improved completeness of orders. Although it wasn't designed to eliminate illegible orders, we actually saw improvement in that area as well." Figure 5-2 shows the reduction in incomplete and illegible orders over the study period.

Home-grown automation

The next step was to eliminate handwritten orders. A home-grown computer program for order entry, created a few years earlier, had never really taken off. The information includes up-to-date lists of LifeCare Hospitals of Pittsburgh physician staff members, patients, and the formulary. The improvement team believed this system could be useful, and two physicians agreed to try it.

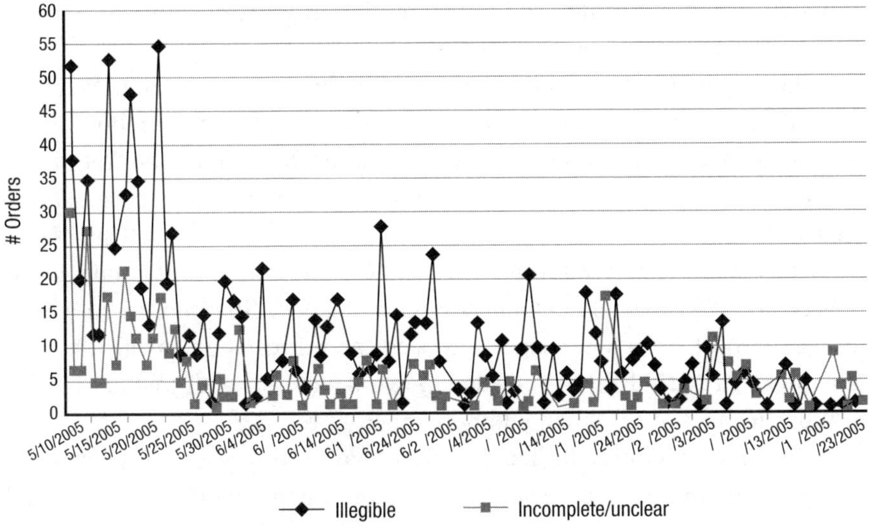

Figure 5-2. Illegible and Incomplete/unclear Orders Decline at LifeCare Hospital.

Coming to the program with differing degrees of computer expertise, the physicians needed varying degrees of one-on-one coaching to become conversant with the ordering system. As they learned to use it, they called for help as needed, and the team responded with real-time problem solving.

Troubleshooting techniques taught by PRHI and reinforced by paid consultants[3] helped the staff quickly identify and remedy the initial problems or "growing pains," and the team anticipates further reduction in illegible and incomplete orders.

Improving the pharmacy

The pharmacy itself was the focus of a three-month improvement effort with the goal of reducing waste and inefficiency and freeing time for the pharmacy technicians. At first, two technicians needed one shift apiece per week to order pharmaceuticals from outside suppliers. The ordering

3. Consultants from Pittsburgh-based Value Capture assisted with the pharmacy work at LifeCare. PRHI supplied education through its Perfecting Patient Care University.

method was cumbersome and inefficient, the drug list incomplete, and the restocking amounts poorly understood.

Starting in 2002, Schreiber led an effort to understand the inventory needed and reduce unnecessary supply. This resulted in a reduction in pharmacy inventory of about one-third between 2002 and 2004. Yet inventory excesses and stock-outs—running out of needed items—occasionally recurred.

Convinced that "reducing inventory" was not the ultimate goal, Schreiber worked to understand the current need. She purchased a customized report on actual usage, and used the information to calculate (1) how much of each drug was needed to avoid stock-outs, (2) which vendor to order from, and (3) when and how much to reorder.

Pharmacy technicians Debbie Reichbaum and Sherry Miller took charge of the project. The result is a *kanban* system, another Toyota-based principle for organizing the timing and flow of supplies. *Kanban* cards contain all necessary information for reorder: vendor, contact information, amount to order, and so forth. These cards are placed at a "trigger" point in the inventory, when enough product remains for a specified number of days—leaving more than enough time to replenish the stock. When the trigger point is reached, the worker removes the *kanban* and places it in the specified bin. Every 24 hours, the *kanbans* are collected and orders are placed. As they went from item to item in the pharmacy creating *kanbans*, Reichbaum and Miller discovered some items long unused, and some of insufficient quantity. Adjusting the amounts required research and intuition.

"Many customizations were required," said Schreiber. "But now, the technicians order every day as part of their regular work. Having the entire pharmacy on a *kanban* system has freed up 16 hours of technician time. My happy dilemma is going to be choosing what to do with that 16 hours, and in this case, we will be expanding our problem-solving capacity."

The number of stock-outs (running out of an item) and other problems has been so greatly reduced that now, each problem that arises can be examined and solved quickly, in real time. The pathway for orders—from the physician's pen to the patient's bedside—is being continuously examined at LifeCare for improvements. Clear and complete orders, a reliable supply of medications, and a way to solve problems in real time every day are key to everyone's work every day.

• SECTION 2 •

IDENTIFYING EVERY PATIENT

"Why are you asking me whether I'm John Smith? I've known you since you were a kid!"

In a small-town like Grove City, Pennsylvania, served by a 95-bed hospital, employees and patients are neighbors and friends. In a place where everyone knows everyone, the common safety practice of checking wristbands to confirm patients' identities strikes some as absurd.

But it's not.

Nurse Kimberle Barker, BSN, RN, knew from an experience earlier in her career how easily mistakes in patient identification happen—even in a larger community, at a bigger hospital and, one that indeed used wristbands.

Mistaken identity is a major problem in hospitals—one that regulators, insurance companies, and hospital boards all want addressed. By chance, Barker had seen how such a mistake could happen: A patient scheduled for cardiac catheterization at an institution where she once worked almost underwent cataract surgery because he had picked up registration and consent forms that were waiting for someone with a similar name. When Barker looked at his band and called him by name, they both realized the dreadful medical error that had almost happened.

That kind of near miss, not to mention an actual error, was the last thing Barker wanted to see happen again.

"Nurses who commit medication errors, or have some part in other mishaps, suffer terribly," says Barker. "You can't imagine how devastating it is when you go into a profession to help people, and end up potentially harming someone."

NURSE NAVIGATOR TRAINING

Barker was one of nine nurses in the Pittsburgh region awarded Nurse Navigator grants through the Jewish Healthcare Foundation. Each Nurse Navigator was given training in the PPC University, and the host institution was given a stipend to pay for some of the nurse's time as he or she embarked on an improvement project. PRHI trainer Debra Thompson, MSN, RN, acted as on-site coach during the year of work with the Navigators, helping with problem solving and training the nurses in on-site data collection as well.

After her initial training, Barker trained others at Grove City in how to make formal observations to see how breakdowns happen. It came down to ID bands. Not every patient always had one. Requisite ID checks were not always done (Figure 5-3 and Table 5-1.) A significant source of resistance was the patients themselves: in small-town America, "You know me," still equals ID.

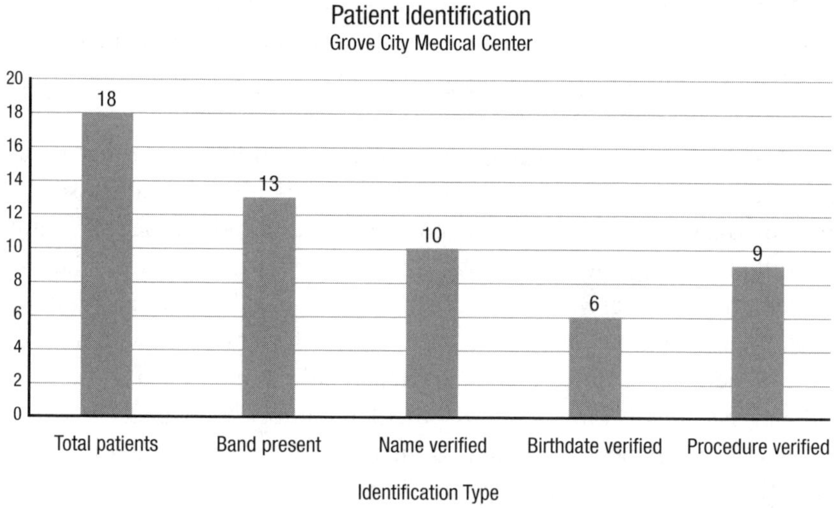

Figure 5-3. Preintervention Observations.

Table 5-1. Pre-intervention Banding and ID Check Rates.

Pre-intervention Banding and ID Check Rates	
Band present	72 percent of the time
Name verified	55 percent
Birth date verified	33 percent
Procedure verified	50 percent

Barker knew that communication—both internal and external—would prove critical to the effort. She gained support from hospital administration for ID banding of all patients, without exception. Barker conducted 29 information sessions for the hospital's 300 employees. The sessions, introduced by the CEO or vice president, were mandatory.

The hospital's communications department began encouraging stories and placing announcements in local newspapers, letting residents know the reason for the new rule, preparing them for the day their neighbor (who's their nurse at the hospital) might enter their room, check that band and ask, "Are you John Smith?" (Figure 5-4)

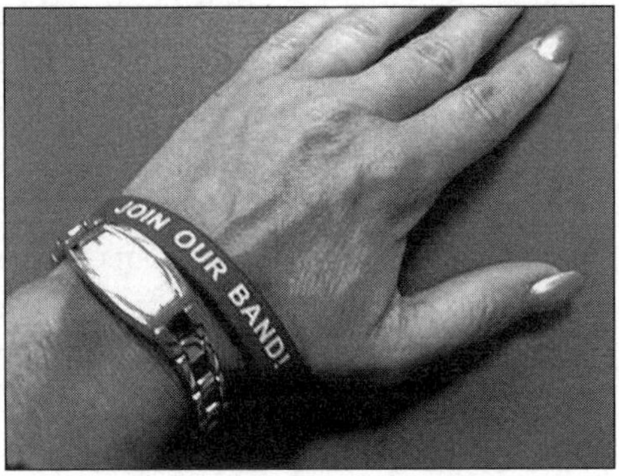

Figure 5-4. Communication was key to the effort. Visual reminders built support for the work.

Banding and active identification of all patients before medications and procedures began in late June 2006. The latest observation showed banding compliance at 100 percent. Medication errors due to misidentification, as expected, are way down (Table 5-2).

"Having support from all the work pathways in the hospital—from the Board to the CEO to Communications—led to broad acceptance by the staff and community," said Barker.

Table 5-2. Reductions in Medication Errors Follow 100 percent Banding Efforts.

Reductions in Medication Errors Follow 100 percent Banding Efforts	
Time period	Number of medication errors related to patient identification
Jan–Dec. 2005	7
June–Sept. 2006	1

• SECTION 3 •

SECRET OF DEPLOYING HIGH-TECH MACHINES: PEOPLE FIRST

It may sound amusing now, but full deployment of the barcode medication administration (BCMA) system at the VA Pittsburgh Healthcare System required the services of a plumber. Now that 99 percent of patients on the 4 West postsurgical unit are receiving their medications on time, the team members there believe they have some crucial information to share about BCMA implementation: Even the most promising, sophisticated electronic systems must be run by real people.

The VA health system won acclaim when, five years ago, it made a massive investment in patient safety by converting to electronic medical records, computerized physician order entry, and BCMA nationwide. The state-of-the-art electronic system, properly and fully deployed, ensures a dramatic improvement in the "five rights" of medication delivery: right patient, right medication, right dose, right time, and right route (oral, IV, etc.). The system automatically tracks every step of the process without adding to the workload of the healthcare professional. Automatic collection of these data quickly makes problems visible, which is the first step toward fixing them.

This sophisticated electronic equipment, however, must be operated by frontline healthcare workers with varying degrees of interest and aptitude. Therein lies the opportunity for designing the way work is done.

Infection project leads to BCMA

Shortly after beginning a project to eliminate antibiotic-resistant infection in the postsurgical unit on 4 West, staff identified the BCMA system as the leading opportunity to eliminate wasted time. In addition to saving time, however, staff members also knew that proper antibiotic administration was crucial, not only in treating antibiotic-resistant MRSA, but in preventing it.

Using the Five Whys, the team learned that the BCMA system broke down every shift because the batteries would run down. Training had not addressed the machine's routine requirements.

Troubleshooting began

The first order of business was to place cue cards on the machine, to ensure that both the computer and scanner batteries were swapped through the charger on a regular schedule. The team posted brief instructions, regarding the simple steps nurses should take to recover from a breakdown. If following the instructions didn't work, then there was a way to call for help. Gone were the days of a nurse puzzling over a malfunctioning machine for 45 minutes.

Enter the plumber

When that was fixed, one mystery still remained: Batteries did not always charge in the charger. Again, the team observed the comings and goings around the machine and discovered the problem. The BCMA battery charger was located next to a sink. When workers washed their hands at the sink, the high water pressure caused water to splash on the electrical outlet, triggering the ground fault interrupter, a safety device that shuts off the outlet in the presence of moisture. A dead outlet meant dead batteries.

Enter the plumber. The water pressure was reduced to keep the water from splashing, an adjustment ultimately made in all the patient rooms in the hospital.

Targeting the training

Once these initial problems were observed and addressed, the team looked at the training gap. Nurses began keeping a log of the problems they encountered, and the team leader tracked calls to the help desk. The training was targeted specifically to the needs expressed.

"Getting used to a whole new way of dispensing medications was a big culture change," says Sharon Parson, RN, the nurse manager on 4 West. "Not every user had the same ability to use this system."

The team identified the stronger users, those with higher-than-average interest and aptitude for using the system. They encouraged any user with a BCMA question or problem to find help through a charge nurse. The BCMA Staff Help Cards on each machine were also helping. (Figure 5-5.).

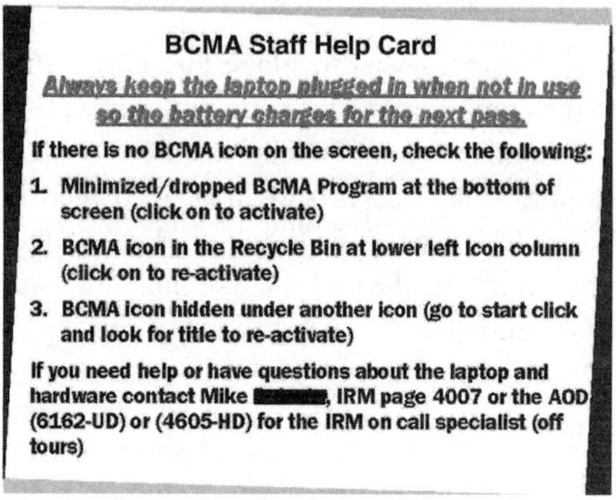

BCMA Staff Help Card

Always keep the laptop plugged in when not in use so the battery charges for the next pass.

If there is no BCMA icon on the screen, check the following:

1. **Minimized/dropped BCMA Program at the bottom of screen (click on to activate)**
2. **BCMA icon in the Recycle Bin at lower left icon column (click on to re-activate)**
3. **BCMA icon hidden under another icon (go to start click and look for title to re-activate)**

If you need help or have questions about the laptop and hardware contact Mike [redacted], IRM page 4007 or the AOD (6162-UD) or (4605-HD) for the IRM on call specialist (off tours)

Figure 5-5. The BCMA Staff Help Card includes simple-to-follow troubleshooting instructions, and somebody to call if problems persist.

90 percent is good: 99 percent is better

Initially, the unit achieved an impressive 90 percent rate of medication timeliness on 4 West. That is, 90 percent of the time, the right patient received the right medication in the right dose within the agreed-upon window of time. "Missing meds," the bane of existence for nurse and pharmacist, were already fairly rare.

But what did 90 percent mean, exactly? Staff delivers between 400 to 600 medications per day to the unit's 30 patients. With 10 percent of the

What Does 90% Mean?

Chances are, hospital and board leaders would be thrilled to learn of a unit where 90 percent of medications were delivered on time. This was the starting point on the 4 West postsurgical unit at the VAPHS.

But what did 90 percent really mean? Of the 400 to 600 doses dispensed on the unit each day, 40 to 60 were late.

"It's hard get to the bottom of 40 or 50 individual problems," says Nurse Manager Sharon Parson.

With 99 percent of medications on time, as they are on most days now, the three or four remaining problems can be solved to root cause in real time, every day.

medications delivered outside the time window, it meant that the nurse leaders would need to follow up on between 40 and 60 doses.

The group began weekly meetings with the pharmacy, troubleshooting things that had gone wrong, patient by patient, one by one. They discovered that, in fixing the root cause of one individual error, they usually solved whole strings of problems that had been plaguing the system. Improvements have continued over time with the rate of medication timeliness on 4 West rising to 99 percent, where it remains (Figure 5-6).

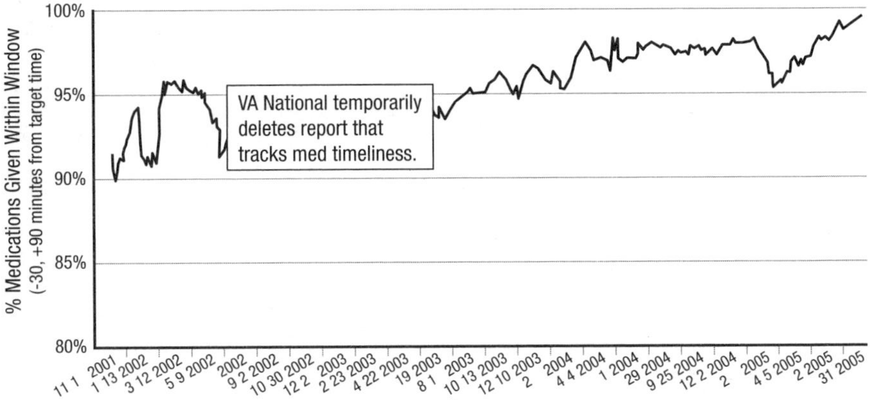

Figure 5-6. The VAPHS Main Hospital Inpatient Surgery Unit: 30-day Moving Average Medications Delivered Within Window.

"Today we might only have two or three medications per day falling outside the window," says Parson. "Now we can really drill down to root cause on each one of those. Usually we find the problem is due to something like the patient's being off the floor for a procedure. Missing medications are extremely rare, thanks to our communication with the pharmacy."

Now the staff knows how they are doing. Parson sends the latest updated on-time medication administration chart with a change-of-shift report, along with other measures of improvement, and posts them on a wall. But nurses do not need to wait: They can get a printout at the end of each medication pass that shows whether or not all of their medications were delivered on time. If they have a problem, they can call for help and continue to care for patients.

Sophisticated electronic machinery can indeed make patients much safer. However, using the machinery to its fullest requires the creativity, commitment, and discipline of the people who do the work.

CHAPTER 6

Eliminating the Wait

CASE STUDIES

- **Section 1. Streamlining the Ambulatory Surgery Center "as quality permits."** The Ambulatory Surgery Center at The Western Pennsylvania Hospital implemented improvements as fast as they could go, but no faster than quality permitted. Patient dignity was at the forefront.
- **Section 2. Let's eliminate the waiting room.** Why should patients wait? Why should they be asked the same question over and over? Looking at processes from the patient's point of view led to improvements at West Penn's Ambulatory Surgery Center.
- **Section 3. Eliminating "Code Red" at a hospital emergency room.** The Emergency Room at Forbes Hospital applied for an "Extreme Makeover" from the quality chief, and got one. Staff and patients were the beneficiaries.
- **Section 4. Getting to the operating room on time in a big-city hospital: the 98.6 percent solution.** Patients were arriving on time in the surgery suite about half the time. Within weeks, almost all of them were. Staff called it the 98.6 percent solution.
- **Section 5. Streamlining intake for children and mentally ill patients.** The most vulnerable patients, children and the mentally ill, shouldn't have to wait for appointments or be delayed upon intake.

Why should patients have to be so patient? Several hospitals across the Pittsburgh region asked themselves why patients had to wait, and received varying—and not very valid—answers. The most stressful situations patients face include coming to the emergency room, coming in for surgery, going through the intake process for a mental-health appointment, or trying to make an appointment for a child thought to have an autistic disorder. At these vulnerable times, waiting only adds anxiety and pressure for patients and staff.

• SECTION 1 •

STREAMLINING THE AMBULATORY SURGERY CENTER "AS QUALITY PERMITS"

Starting to use Perfecting Patient Care requires a commodity that's both rare and counterintuitive in a pressured healthcare system: patience. Experiences with PRHI's partners have revealed something else that seems counterintuitive: It's okay to start small. Theorists speculate that the only successful application will take place when an entire institution, wall to wall, has bought into the concept and is willing to do business an entirely different way. While striving for this ideal condition may be a good place to start, the experiments in Pittsburgh have shown that small pilots can also lead to transformation. Starting small—a small unit, just a few beds, one or two "minor" problems—can help an organization get to the starting gate. However, whether a pilot is large or small, wide adoption of the principles relies on culture change in the organization, emanating from top leadership.

During the first few months on the Ambulatory Surgery Center (ASC) at West Penn in early 2002, the entire staff, team leader Gloria Teichman, RN, and teachers supplied by PRHI, began making several process improvements. But a more dramatic story was under way: New knowledge took hold that change was possible.

Once staff members saw that calling out problems led to their ultimate solution, more and more people reported more and more problems. Teichman saw the hope: Staff members felt as though they had what they needed to actually fix what was wrong. Keeping up with the new, heightened expectations became the real challenge.

Ramping up "as quality permits"

America's fast-paced culture creates expectations of instant results, and wide, fast dissemination of new ideas. In a typical American industry, management is usually asked to achieve full production as soon as possible—volume first, quality second.

Perfecting Patient Care, like any Toyota-based system of work redesign, requires rampup at a more deliberate pace. The focus during startup is on the customer—and that means quality first. Quantity is achieved "as quality permits."

Why go slowly? First is that big prerequisite, culture change, emanating from top management. It requires creating a work environment that's safe emotionally, professionally and physically. Even when the current system isn't working well, people naturally resist change. They need time to learn, understand and adapt to a new way of working.

In his case study on Toyota's Georgetown, Kentucky plant, Harvard professor Kazuhiro Mishina stresses the importance of setting "a deliberately slow rampup schedule."[1] Mishina notes that workers adapting to this new system must learn certain principles and arrive at that eye-opening moment—which varies among individuals—when they fully comprehend how it can work for them in their own environment.

Sometimes the epiphany comes from solving one key problem to root cause—not a "manufactured" problem, but one encountered in the everyday work routine. For example, at the West Penn ASC, workers noticed that patients' waiting times varied a great deal. Over half of the patients were waiting for 1-1/2 hours—some as many as five hours. Yet other patients breezed through the system.

Initial experiments looked at establishing a "signal" from the operating room (OR) back to the ASC—a line of communication where none had existed. When surgeons began the closing procedures for one surgery, which usually takes 45 minutes, a signal would be sent to the patient holding area so that preparations could be properly concluded on the next patient. This experiment was promising: The signal reduced waiting times for four patients from two hours to between 40 and 65 minutes.

But these initial experiments revealed another systemic flaw. Upon arrival, patients were to have blood drawn, so that the lab results would be available in plenty of time for the scheduled surgery. However, when ORs become available, patients might be rushed in ahead of schedule, only to then have to wait for lab results, delaying patient, surgeon, and operating team (Figure 6-1).

---

1. Mishina Kazuhiro, Toyota Motor Manufacturing, U.S.A., Inc., Harvard Business School Case # 693019, (September 8, 1992).

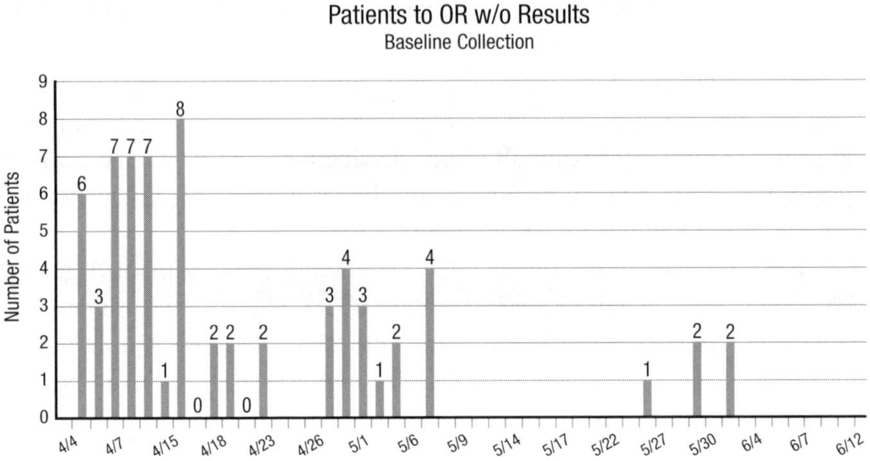

Figure 6-1. The number of patients arriving in the OR without lab results went to zero, once the communications and supply-line issues were addressed.

The team concluded that the signal for drawing blood must be a well-understood part of the pathway. It must be done before the patient enters the holding area, in a reliable location—a room dedicated to pre-op blood draws.

A supply closet was converted into a blood draw room, based on the phlebotomist's detailed specifications and understanding of the work pathway (Figure 6-2). Patients began to have their blood drawn immediately after registration. While the patient awaits the signal from the operating room, the lab processes the results.

Unraveling the cause of a single problem can lead in unanticipated directions. Reducing patients' waiting time revealed underlying problems with OR timing, lab scheduling, physical space, and sequencing of the work. Fixing a small problem to its root cause had the unexpected "side effect" of fixing several larger, systemic problems.

Problems hiding in plain sight

A new physician on staff noticed a busy hallway in the ASC between the waiting room and the surgical prep area with beds. Patients sat, lined up in the chairs, dressed in hospital gowns, sometimes for an hour or more,

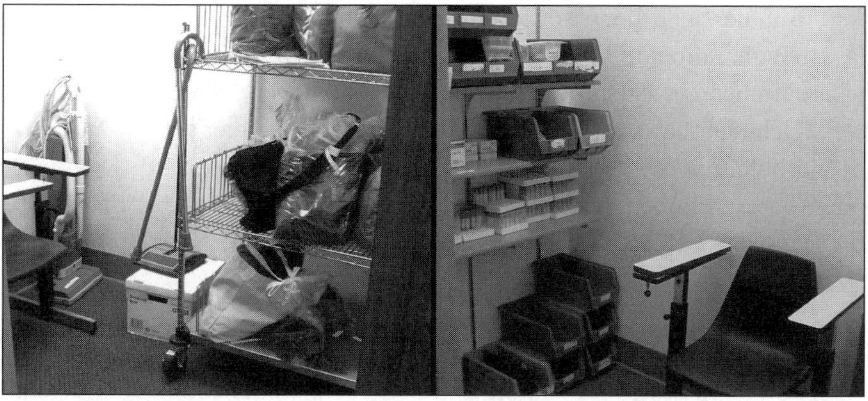

Figure 6-2. *Before* and *after*: supply closet transformed to blood draw area. Left, before. Right, after disciplined 5S process and knowledge of the worker about what was needed for the patient.

waiting to be assigned to a bed. When a bed in the surgical prep area became available, the patient would move from chair to bed. The new physician alerted the team leader to the problem.

"We'd been using the chairs to 'store' patients for 20 years," said Teichman. "We wanted to be sure they were ready. But we realized nobody who works here ever had to sit in the chairs. Once we really looked at it from the patients' point of view, we wanted to fix it immediately."

The team of administrative assistants and nurses set out to find a solution. They realized that the system relied on "pushing" patients into waiting areas, rather than waiting for the "pull" of bed availability. The team devised a system where the charge nurse in the surgical prep area would call the secretary as a bed became available.

Initial reluctance within the team gave way to, "We might as well try it tomorrow."

In a matter of hours, the experiment was deemed a success. Since that day, no patient has sat in the hallway in a hospital gown. Waiting time decreased; scheduling efficiency increased.

As team leader, Teichman actually learned the work of the secretary, the receptionist, and the chart maker, in an attempt to understand the interactions or pathways in the work flow. She discovered how easy a job looks, until you try to do it yourself.

To understand how work is done, Teichman took "field trips" to the lab, to registration, to scheduling, and even to the print shop—some places where, in her 22 years at the hospital, she had never visited.

Teichman and the team learned to view one another's work and each new problem with new eyes. The result was a more respectful workplace, one where calling out problems became an expectation and an opportunity for teamwork.

Honor Nurses by Saving Their Time

Chart builders assemble elaborate charts for patients coming in for surgery. These charts contain all necessary forms for patient, hospital, insurance, and physician. Every single form in the chart must be stamped beforehand with the patient's identifying information. If a form is not stamped, a nurse in the presurgery area is usually the one to discover it. Before the improvement work began in the ASC, it was the nurse who had to take apart the chart, stamp the blank page, then reassemble the chart—two minutes, ten seconds of nursing time per chart, which translated to over an hour a day of RN time.

Once they realized it was a problem, the chart builders made a few simple changes in the course of their work that almost eliminated the problem (Figure 6-3). Charts will soon be delivered to the RNs 100 per-

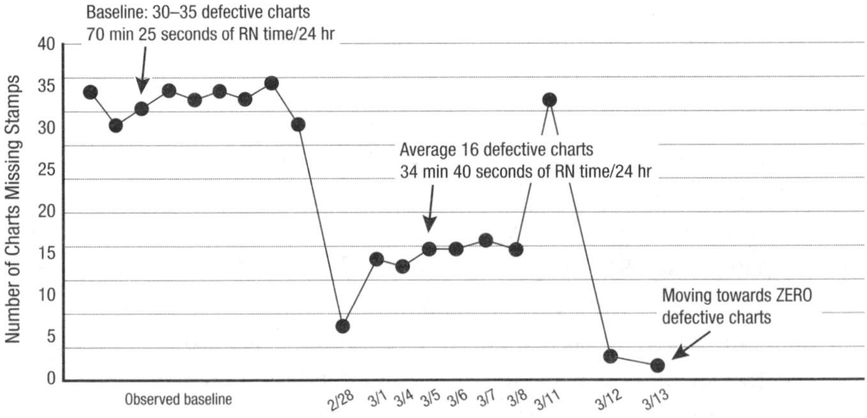

Figure 6-3. Stamping Out Defective Charts Through Wall-to-wall Communication.

cent stamped and defect free. The new system will make it impossible to deliver a defective chart.

The results save over six hours per week of nursing time and have increased job satisfaction for both nurses and chart builders.

Contagion—the good kind

As Team Leader Teichman noticed after six months of Perfecting Patient Care experiments, problem solving became contagious among the staff. By focusing on what patients need, the team created:

- A more compassionate patient experience through:
  - Reducing waiting times.
  - Eliminating hallway chairs as waiting spots.
  - Using comfortable recliners in the preevaluation area instead of uninviting tables (Figure 6-4).

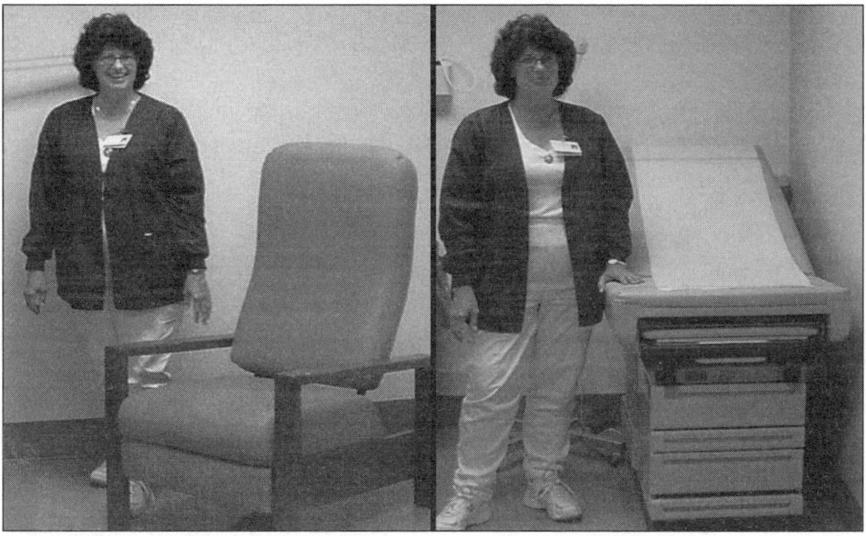

Figure 6-4. Increasing Patient Dignity. After locating several unused recliners in other areas of the hospital, ASC nurses used them to replace the cold, uninviting tables in the evaluation area. Here, Mary Shane, RN, shows the result. Patients vastly prefer meeting their healthcare team members from these comfortable, dignified chairs.

- A more compassionate work place by:
  - Expanding the desk area.
  - Reducing duplicative work.
  - Streamlining processes for physician orders and history and physicals.
  - Organizing supplies and locating them more conveniently.

When courageous hospital leaders focus on deliberate rampup, insisting on quality for each patient and healthcare worker before wider dissemination, success is contagious and sustainable.

New "Eyes to See" Reveal Problem and Solution

The postoperative area for the ASC is a short-stay recovery unit with seven beds. However, one of these scarce bed areas was completely consumed by supplies. The team leader, Gloria Teichman, RN, discovered that the space was virtually overrun with boxes of gynecological pads. It was time to ask a few "Whys."

Why weren't they on the storage shelves? Because it, too, was full of boxes of pads. A nurse informed Teichman, "We have more boxes stored down the hall in the bathroom."

In all, 3,588 pads—a generous year's supply—were stored on the floor, with more arriving all the time. Teichman discovered that the pads were not being deliberately ordered, but had been placed on "auto order," leaving workers to scurry around to find more storage spaces.

Teichman suspended the auto order, returned many of the boxes, and effectively turned off what had become a perpetual motion. All seven beds in the recovery unit are now ready to accept patients.

• SECTION 2 •

LET'S ELIMINATE THE WAITING ROOM

Once the West Penn Ambulatory Surgery Center (ASC) began using Perfecting Patient Care to phase in improvements, a number of big gains had already been made. And while the wait time had been fluctuating between 1-1/2 hours and five hours, patients still waited as much as an hour during registration. At the beginning of the experiments, an hour's wait would have looked like a victory. Now it looked like another opportunity for improvement. Patients seem resigned to the "fact" that waiting is part of healthcare—it certainly isn't usually defined as a problem needing a solution. Yet for patients facing surgery, the waiting can provoke needless and harmful anxiety. Some get frustrated and leave.

Given new "eyes to see," seven registration team members at West Penn's ASC realized that, despite advances in registration and lab times, waiting continued to be a problem for patients.

The team probed more deeply, "Why can't we just eliminate waiting time?" They decided to work together toward a more ideal condition.

Repetition = waste

The only reason a patient needs to be present to register at all is to sign consents and receive an ID bracelet. It should take only moments. Part of the problem was that during registration, team members found themselves asking patients for missing personal information. For the most part, patients had already given this information by phone to another department in advance. A connection was broken: Information received in one department was not making its way to the chart at registration.

As is often the problem in a large, complex organization, the root cause of this registration problem lay in another department. Especially where a lean "experiment" may be going on in one department, but not another, top leaders may need to intervene to ensure each department gets the needed information, supplies, and cooperation. In this case, workers in the other department became engaged and quickly devised solutions for their "customers," the registration clerks. With correct personal patient information on every chart every time, registration time got shorter. Further refinements led to even more improvements in the work flow.

"Why can't we do even better?"

Although the time it took to register each patient dropped dramatically (Figure 6-5), the goal of the registration clerks had not yet been met: eliminating the time patients have to wait.

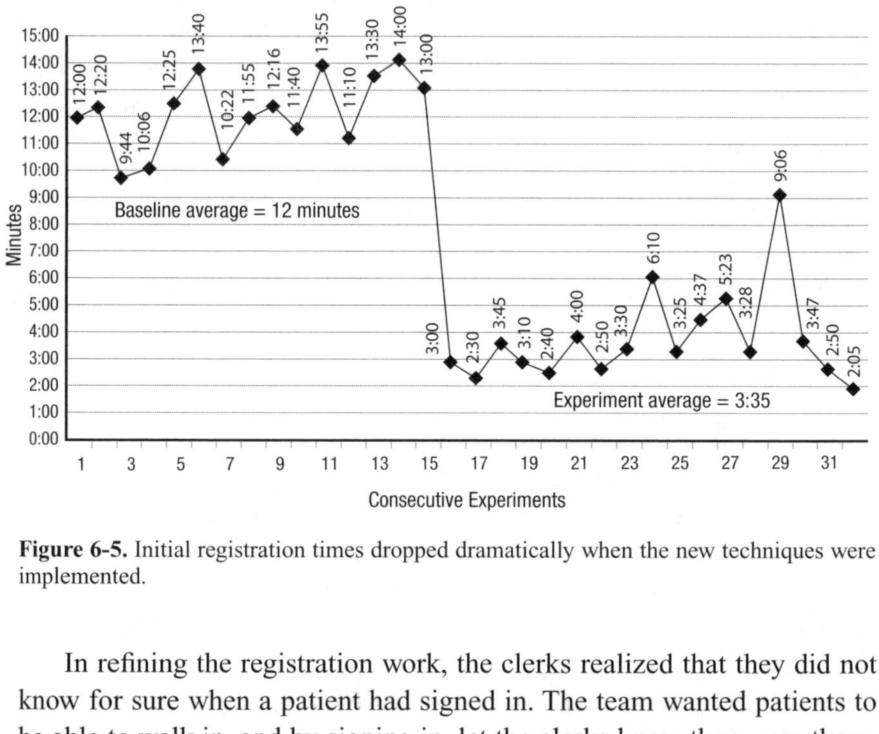

Figure 6-5. Initial registration times dropped dramatically when the new techniques were implemented.

In refining the registration work, the clerks realized that they did not know for sure when a patient had signed in. The team wanted patients to be able to walk in, and by signing in, let the clerks know they were there. They tried numerous experiments—always including patients in their tests—before arriving at a redesign that worked. It involved an inexpensive plastic item from the office store and a color coding system (Figure 6-6, photos A, B, and C).

The experiment cannot be said to be "done," because further refinements are always under way. However, patient wait times have dropped

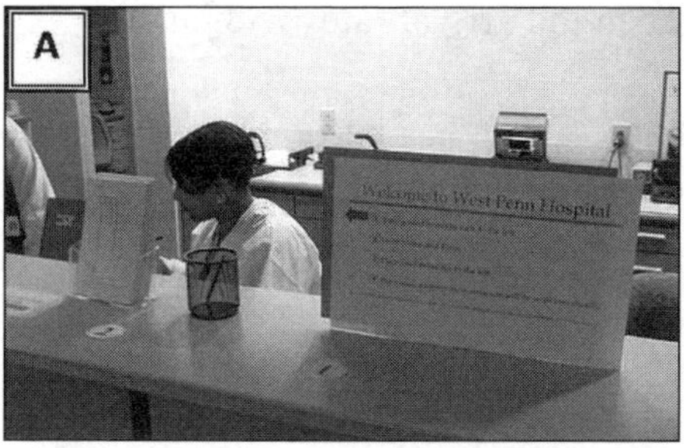

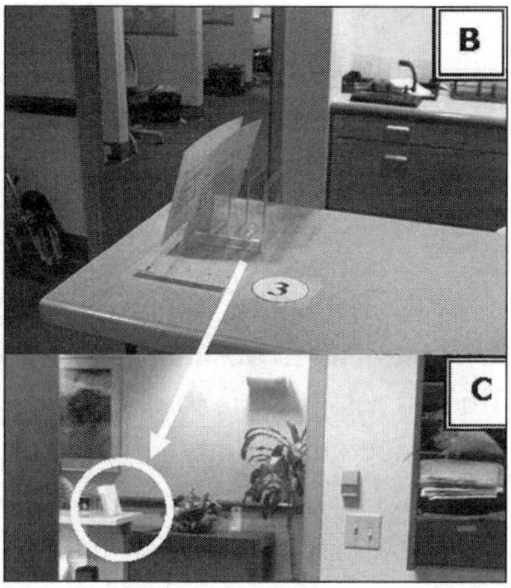

Figure 6-6. A. clear, color-coded instructions greet patients. In fact, patients willingly participated in experiments to improve wait times, and their input helped staff improve the system based on patient needs. **B.** An inexpensive plastic holder places bright yellow cards upright, creating a visual cue. **C.** from where the registration clerk sits. Through various modifications, the system is still in use three years later.

dramatically, and the changes have been sustained for a year (Figure 6-7). The most significant improvements were:

- Patients are no longer waiting 45 minutes to an hour to have pretesting completed.

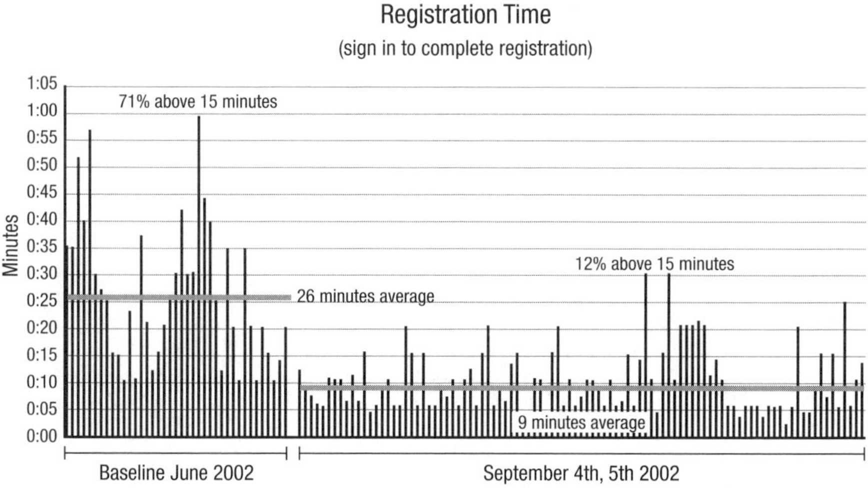

Figure 6-7. Total registration times remained down following implementation of new procedures.

- Staff can handle volume surges in the arrival rates without any significant problems.
- With stable timing established, the group has been able to focus on other changes aimed at an even more efficient flow through the preoperative pathway.

PRHI coach, David Sharbaugh, said, “When people get frustrated in their daily work because the system makes it hard to be successful, the traditional response is to blame it on the system, the management, or to just disengage and simply come to work and ‘do your job.’ Perfecting Patient Care, above all else, is about helping people to be successful in meaningful work. When workers begin to make small changes in their own work, they realize that they can change the system. Imagine 2,500 employees, every day, making small changes that help better meet patient needs, eliminate waste, improve flow, and increase productivity.”

One team member put it succinctly: “I don’t ever want to go back to doing it the old way!”

• SECTION 3 •

ELIMINATING "CODE RED" AT A HOSPITAL EMERGENCY ROOM

Healthcare improvement experts call it the "current condition"—that unvarnished assessment of a situation that currently exists. An honest, uncritical assessment of the current condition can prove eye opening, even painful, but is essential to mapping the way for improvement. In July 2006, the current condition at the emergency room (ER) at West Penn Allegheny Hospital's Forbes Campus was less than ideal.

Ambulances were being diverted from the ER about 60 hours a month, meaning that up to 200 patients were being taken to other hospitals because of a lack of available beds. The diversion status, called Code Red, means longer ambulance rides for patients, and up to $3 million in lost revenue for the hospital.

Once in the ER, patients might have to wait for hours to be seen, formally admitted, and transferred to a room in an appropriate unit. While "boarding" in the ER, these patients may not have received optimal care for their conditions, since emergency medicine is a separate clinical discipline from inpatient care.

Patient satisfaction scores for the ER experience were disappointing, although staff members perceived that they were working harder than ever.

Forbes was not alone. Hospitals across the country report that crowded emergency rooms are necessitating more diversions. The reasons include both *supply*—fewer available, staffed beds[2]—and *demand*—more people seeking treatment in the nation's ERs. Some hospitals are adding ER beds, but others are looking at the bigger picture for answers. Larger gains, they believe, can be made by looking at the way patients flow through the entire hospital—finding and using all beds, for example, and streamlining appropriate discharges.

---

2. A staffed bed refers to a bed in a unit that has an adequate number of nurses on the shift. One consequence of the current nursing shortage is that empty beds may exist, but not enough nurses are available to tend to additional patients. (See a fuller discussion of the consequences of the nursing shortage in Chapter 2, Section 3.)

At Forbes, all of these approaches are occuring simultaneously: As the ER is remodeled and expanded, from the current 16 beds to 25, the entire hospital staff is looking for ever more creative ways to use every bed they have.

Extreme team

"The first thing we came to understand was that this was not an ER problem, but a hospital problem" says Diane Frndak, Vice President for Quality with the West Penn Allegheny Health System, expert in Toyota-based system improvements, and former coach and education expert for PRHI. "These aren't ER patients, they're everyone's patients. It's a very complex problem, and we need everyone's brain to help untangle it and make it better for patients."

The untangling began in June when staff members across the hospital were invited to become self-appointed members of the "Extreme Team," designing an extreme makeover for the ER. For one week, a room paneled with white poster boards became the brainstorming zone. Any person on the hospital staff who had an idea and wrote it on a poster board received a free piece of pizza. Hundreds of ideas began to accumulate—varied, innovative, unusual but most of all, feasible.

Even more important, staff members who *actually tried a new idea* received an Extreme Team T-shirt.

"Some people thought pizza and T-shirts were corny or undignified, but for the vast majority, it was an unexpectedly fun way to build a team. Most important, we were unundated with ideas. We still have some ideas from those poster boards to try," said Frndak, "but try them we will. It's inspired us to make a lot of rapid-cycle improvements."

Team members began to observe work in various areas of the hospital to develop a frank understanding of the current condition. They observed for 12 hours on each floor, with an eye toward streamlining communications (bed locations and status, movement of patients from unit to unit) and processes (quicker admissions and discharges). They looked respectfully at processes as a way to learn: The observations involved no blame.

They began to uncover system problems and ask:

- Where are the vacant beds? How can we communicate quickly that a discharge has occurred?
- How can we make the discharge faster while giving more complete information to each patient?
- Processing a new patient on the floor takes a nurse an hour. Is there any way to make this process more efficient?

Rapid-cycle improvements

The observations and posted ideas formed the basis for rapid-cycle improvements. Angela Henzler, RN, director, emergency services and team leader said, "We became one big team. If a patient was on a gurney in the ER hallway, we immediately formed a huddle, redesigned the process, perhaps tried one of the new ideas, but solved the problem on the spot. The benefits were great for patients, but also for staff. We developed trust and now we work so well together—all in the interest of the patient."

Twice a day, for 10 or 15 minutes, Extreme Team members—staffing specialists, a representative from each unit, bed allocators, housekeepers, and others—convene for a "bed meeting." Together they quickly discuss how many beds are available on each unit, how many of those beds are staffed, whether a charge nurse is on duty, how many patients are currently on the unit, how many beds are open, how many discharge orders are pending, and how many additional discharges are possible. Other considerations include how many new patients have just been moved to the unit, and how many are due to transfer.

By offering everyone a snapshot of the entire hospital, along with an idea of where the bottlenecks are likely to develop, the bed meetings replace suspicion and competition among units with camaraderie. By eliminating silos, reaction moves from "It's not my problem" to "How can I help?"

The meetings also uncover other problems. For example, one unit was out of orange armbands for patients at risk for falling. They devised an experiment to first get armbands immediately where needed, and then figure out how to redesign the system to keep from running out again.

Moving patients from one unit to another, and bringing a new patient up from the ED are time-consuming processes for unit nurses. The patients must be assessed and information gathered and put into the computer. The bed meeting is one way to try to coordinate these movements so that no single unit is overwhelmed.

Staff members experimented with other ways to avoid overwhelming units with new admissions. They standardized a checklist to produce a defect-free admission. Then, by reallocating time, one nurse was freed up to become the "admissions nurse," using the checklist to perform the initial assessment and computer entry, while the patient is still in the ED. The admissions nurse reduces the initial workload for the unit nurse and improves the quality of information and efficiency of the handoff. With a checklist accompanying each patient, each step is sure to be completed.

Just in case: contingency plans

Should there be a surge in ER admissions in the next several hours, what is the contingency plan? This question is among those routinely considered at the bed meetings. Staffing specialists discuss who is on call and how such an eventuality could be handled. Before these meetings, plans were too often made under duress during a crisis. Continually anticipating surges in the workload gives the teams an opportunity for buffer options—just in case.

"Every day has its own dynamics," says Henzler. "We are finding new ways every day to share intelligence and improve teamwork."

The results

Since July 2005, almost no Code Reds have been declared at Forbes (Figure 6-8). In fact, the number of ER visits increased by over 1,000 between July and October as compared to budgeted visits. Forbes routinely stabilizes and transports patients in need of services like interventional cardiology, which is offered at the larger Allegheny General Hospital (AGH). In fact, AGH has 34 ER beds, and provided 44,000 visits in the past year. Interestingly, Forbes with its 16 beds and Extreme Team "makeover" has provided 40,000 visits in the past year.

Press-Ganey scores of patient satisfaction have also improved on every shift, for every employee group. Figure 6-9 shows the gains for physicians—a gain that still does not satisfy Adrian D'Amico, MD, who heads the ER. "We won't be happy until our scores exceed 95 percent," said Dr. D'Amico, "and then we'll keep improving."

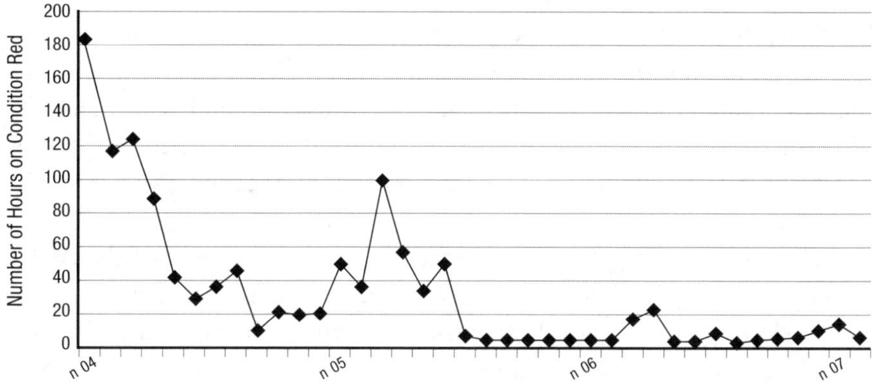

Figure 6-8. Code Red Hours at Forbes Regional Campus from December 2003 Through February 2007.

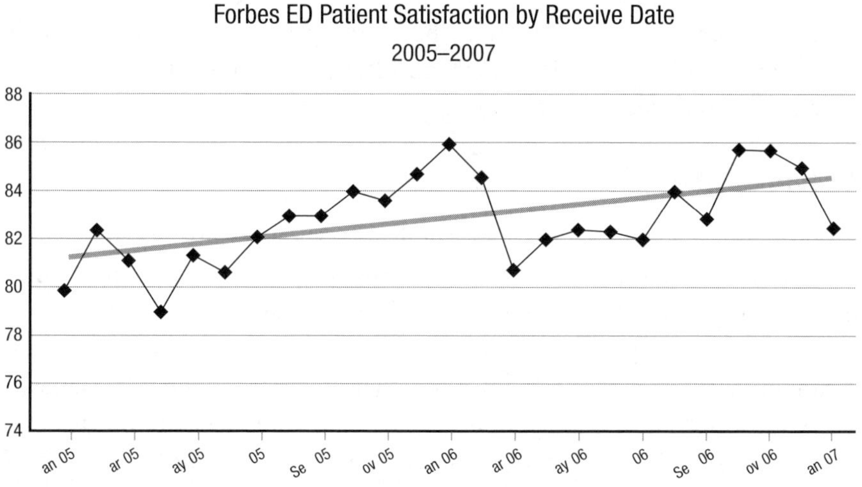

Figure 6-9. Patient Satisfaction Scores Show Corresponding Rise.

• SECTION 4 •

GETTING TO THE OPERATING ROOM ON TIME IN A BIG-CITY HOSPITAL: THE 98.6 PERCENT SOLUTION

Staff members in the Ambulatory Care Center (ACC) at Allegheney General Hospital took off running with Perfecting Patient Care, and quickly improved patient flow. Kim Sperring, vice president, and Jean Schmidt, director of peri-operative services, supported the application of this process in the ACC with help from then-on-site PRHI coach, Diane Frndak, and others from PRHI.

The aim is to improve the satisfaction of all customers of the ACC: patients, staff, and physicians. Patients need efficient care; staff needs a steady flow of work; and physicians need their patients to arrive in the operating room on time. It all boils down to meeting patient needs and making employees successful in their work.

The problem was that only 54.5 percent—just over half—of the patients scheduled for surgery arrived in the operating room on time. Physicians were frustrated; staff members and patients were too.

Several employees throughout the working pathway completed Perfecting Patient Care University through PRHI. This preparation seemed to hasten progress once work began.

Waiting for the "pull"

According to Dawn Chiaramonte, RN, Nurse Manager, ACC, patient wait times have decreased by 1 to 1.5 hours by applying a simple "pull" methodology. Pull means that the ACC (upstream process) should not have a patient ready for surgery until the operating room (OR) (downstream process) needs the patient. So, rather than processing all first cases at 5 AM—which caused long waits for patients, bottlenecks in the system, and chaos for staff—patients are now processed according to the time of their surgery and a set of specific priorities.

The priorities are necessary because patients have different needs, and the ACC must be able to predict when they can complete pre-op preparation so as not to delay surgery. Priorities include the need for acute-pain service, testing on the day of surgery, history and physical, and special equipment. Staffing schedules were changed to facilitate patient flow, and to synchronize with the OR. Now they have patients ready when the orderlies from pre-op arrive.

One by one, the small changes, implemented by the people closest to the work, in the interest of the patients, have succeeded. Within just a few weeks of starting the improvement work, the number of cases arriving on time to the OR climbed to 98.5 percent, and remained over 85 percent for a year (Table 6-1). Patients no longer languish in the registration area, either. Most are registered within 10 minutes of arrival (Table 6–2).

Table 6–1. First Cases On Time to the Operating Room at Allegheny General.

First Cases On Time to the Operating Room at Allegheny General	
Nov. 2003, (Beginning PPC)	54.5 percent
June 2004	98.6 percent
Average from Nov. 2003–June 2004	88.6 percent

Table 6-2. Registration Within 10 Minutes of ACC Check-in.

Registration Within 10 Minutes of ACC Check-in	
Before Feb. 2004 (start of PPC)	>10 percent
Feb.–May 2004, average	91.4 percent

Find the Family

After a procedure, physicians would often go to the family waiting room to discuss the outcome with the family, only to discover that the family had just stepped out for a snack.

To improve this connection, the ACC initiated a Patient Contact Sheet that is placed on the front of the patient's chart. It includes the patient name, surgery date, family/significant other name, cell phone number, pager number, and waiting area. This decreases missed connections by giving a specific set of instructions for communicating with families. The ACC now provides a pager for families who request it.

When problems are seen from the patient's point of view, solutions can more readily be found and implemented.

• SECTION 5 •

STREAMLINING INTAKE FOR CHILDREN AND MENTALLY ILL PATIENTS

Patients are inconvenienced by having to wait weeks for a physician appointment. However, for the most vulnerable patients, such as children who may have an autistic disorder, or a person struggling with a mental illness, long waits for appointments can be unacceptable barriers to treatment. Two organizations in the Pittsburgh region have succeeded in reducing wait times for these vulnerable populations.

CHILD DEVELOPMENT UNIT, CHILDREN'S HOSPITAL OF PITTSBURGH OF UPMC

It's usually a long road for parents and children who are finally referred for evaluation for autistic spectrum disorder. Typically, a child will be exhibiting symptoms for months or years, as the family struggles with the effects of the puzzling behavior. The pediatrician eventually refers a child for evaluation to a place like the child development unit (CDU) at Children's Hospital of Pittsburgh of UPMC. This unit specializes in evaluating developmental delays and autistic spectrum disorders. With ambivalence and great anxiety, the parent places that first call.

Before

Before improvements began, the encounter might have gone like this: The parent, in this case, the mother, places the call and lands in voicemail, where she shares a few words about the child's condition and a callback number. The following day a person calls her back. If the mother is out, phone tag can ensue for days.

When they finally meet by phone, the sympathetic intake coordinator asks a series of questions to determine, among other things, if the family's concerns can be addressed by the CDU specialists. If it sounds like the child would be a candidate for CDU evaluation, the intake coordinator sends the parents two questionnaires: one for them, one for the child's teacher. When these forms are completed and sent back, the process will continue.

Weeks usually pass before the parents send the forms back. Meanwhile the child's outbursts may have grown more frequent and intense. Once the intake coordinator reviews the information, he or she recommends the best type of CDU appointment and sends a letter to the parents letting them know they can now call to schedule an appointment. It will be a two-hour appointment, thorough in every way. They will get answers.

At last the mother calls to schedule, only to discover that the first available appointment is 10 weeks away—almost five months from the day she summoned her courage to place the first call. The desperate mother bursts into tears. The frustrated CDU staff member feels like crying too. All involved want to see that child far more quickly.

After

What started as an attempt to address a leader's goal transformed the way appointments are made at the CDU. Leadership of Children's Hospital challenged all units to answer all phone calls live, and to schedule appointments at the time of the parent's first call.

In 2004, the unit's Medical Director, Dr. Robert Noll, along with Project Specialist Tina Hahn and Manager Iris Harlan attended the week-long Perfecting Patient Care University offered by PRHI. The classes illuminated certain techniques for these unit leaders—not so much the "what" but the "how" of improvement. By focusing solely on the needs of each individual patient, they were told, they could streamline processes and make improvements they hadn't thought possible. PRHI's Debra Thompson, MSN, RN, coached the team members as they began experimenting with process improvements.

"The first question we asked was, 'Why can't we answer all calls live? And how can we move closer to that ideal?'" says Thompson. "We didn't start by asking, 'How can we get appointments to happen faster?' Instead, we patiently untangled the problem and started with a manageable chunk at the front end of the whole process."

Staff had been starting off every morning a full day behind on phone calls. Each morning they faced playing back a day's worth of voicemail and calling each person. It never occurred that it could work any other way, since the volume of calls was so great.

Hahn in her role as team leader, made phone calls alongside the intake coordinators until they caught up on the backlog. Within 24 hours, the phones were being answered in real time, with only a few landing in voicemail. Not only did this new process eliminate up to three days of wait time for patients, the intake coordinators discovered that it greatly reduced their stress. The time they'd spent listening to voicemails was put to more productive purposes—answering calls live and reviewing charts. Suddenly, they discovered, the hours in their work day went a lot farther.

Unanticipated results

One unanticipated result of taking the calls live was that the volume of intakes completed rose from 294 to 379, revealing additional facets of the community need for the types of services provided by the CDU (Figure 6-10). It also caused more problems to surface. For example, staff

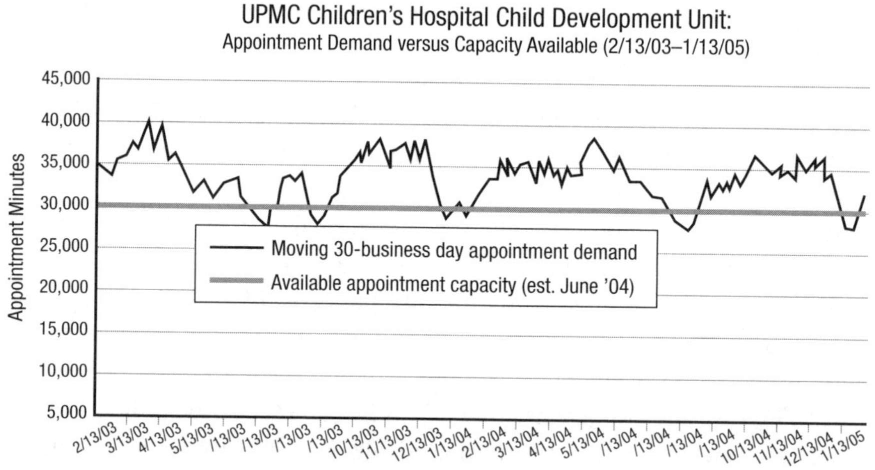

Figure 6-10. Understanding Supply and Demand.

Demand: Once "in the system," parents report a high degree of satisfaction with the services their children receive. The problem is that, since this is the only program of its kind in the region, more demand exists than capacity.

Problems: The lag in capacity was not the only factor that led to waits of four to six months for a first appointment.

Solutions: Continually addressing small, manageable problems, one by one, guided solely by what was in the best interest of the patients, led to breakthroughs over time.

knew that only 60 percent of the people who made the initial call for help actually returned the paperwork and received appointments. Would this percentage improve if staff scheduled the appointment at the time of the call, and then exchanged paperwork? Or would doing so increase the amount of incomplete paperwork or missed appointments? The CDU staff is phasing in the zero-paperwork appointment, currently with patients up to age three.

"Tackling the whole problem of 'wait time' is too overwhelming," says team leader Hahn. "It works better to break it into smaller pieces, like scheduling two-year-olds at time of intake, seeing how that goes, fixing as we go, then expanding that offering. By approaching change in this way, work becomes more manageable. Working this way, and relying on the training we received in the Perfecting Patient Care University, has already allowed us to get better results than we ever thought possible."

With the steps taken thus far, CDU staff has eliminated three days of up-front wait time for all patients by taking calls live (Figure 6-11). Also, children up the age of three are being scheduled at the time of intake, eliminating another component of the wait time for an appointment. The

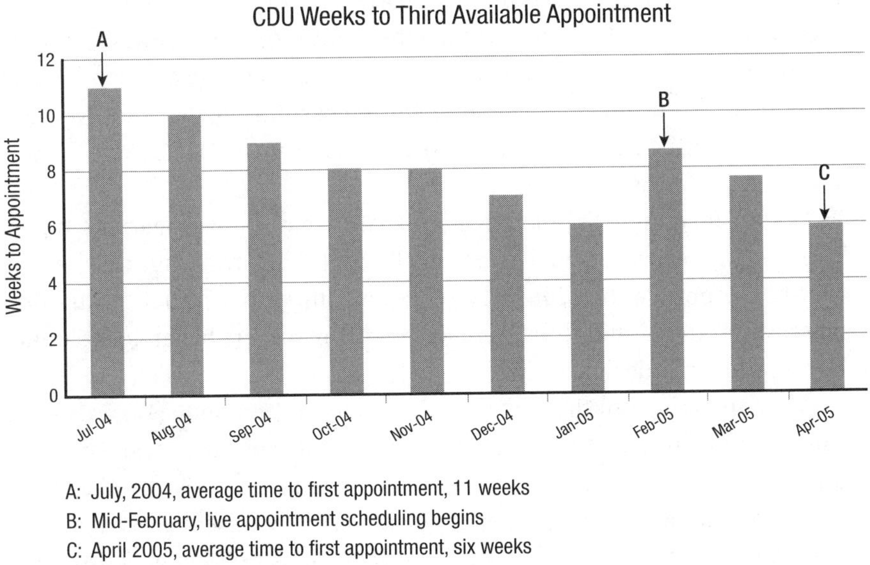

Figure 6-11. Appointment Times Shrink.

plan is to move ahead with small, frequent improvements to ensure children with special needs get exactly what they need when they need it.

According to Dr. Noll, "Our goal for intakes is to have families make one call and get scheduled. Additionally, we believe it is extremely important to see children and their families in a timely manner. One phone call and a timely appointment is our goal for quality family-centered care." The CDU staff continue to look at ways to streamline appointment scheduling, create the ideal appointment to thoroughly assess each patient, and work with the families to design an intervention plan for their children.

FAMILY SERVICES OF WESTERN PENNSYLVANIA STREAMLINES INTAKE

It just didn't add up. Deneen Sobota, RN, knew that when patients came for their first appointments at Family Services of Western Pennsylvania, nurses routinely conducted a thorough mental-health evaluation. And yet, physicians still had to spend time during initial consultations going over questions, clarifying answers, and asking for more information.

"We were getting lots of good information in our evaluations," said Sobota. "But often, it wasn't the information the doctor needed."

Sobota was awarded a Nurse Navigator grant from the Jewish Healthcare Foundation, which offered her team-training and gave a stipend to her employer to buy a little of her time for a year during the improvement work. The grant also provided on-site visits from PRHI coach, Debra Thompson, MSN, RN.

At staff meetings, Sobota began to share what she was learning about process standardization in Perfecting Patient Care training and how it might help improve the efficiency of the all-important initial evaluation. Once reassured that their jobs were safe, staff members began to welcome opportunities to redesign work.

When mapping out the way work had always been done (Figure 6-12), Sobota discovered that nurses jotted down answers to questions they thought the physician needed to know. The lack of a standardized evaluation led to missed information, some of it crucial. Consequently, appointments ran as much as an hour behind, as physicians filled in gaps from the initial patient interviews.

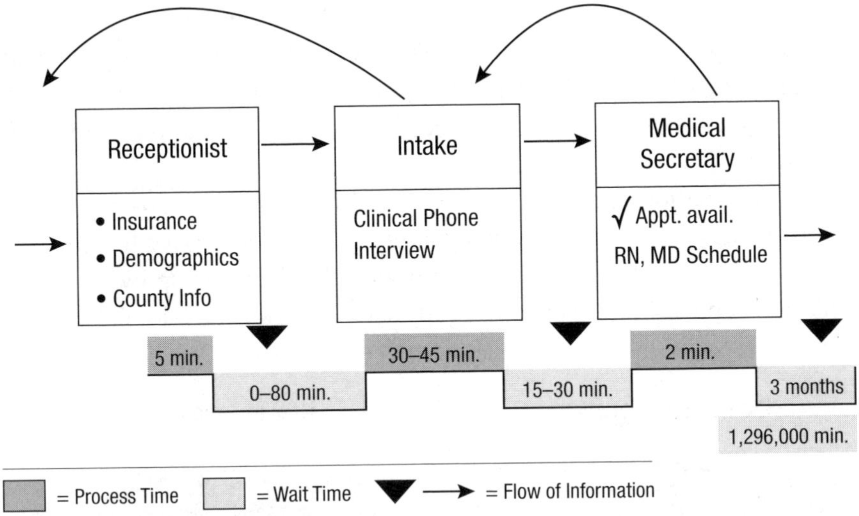

Figure 6-12. Process mapping. Sobota created a process map, showing where time and information were leaking out of the encounter, costing time and fraying nerves of patients and healthcare workers alike.

The team discovered that nurses working with child psychiatrists used a standardized set of intake questions. As a result, those physicians generally had all the background information they needed during the first appointment. With some research, nurses working on the adult-care team found a version of that tool to use on their own evaluations. (Figure 6-13)

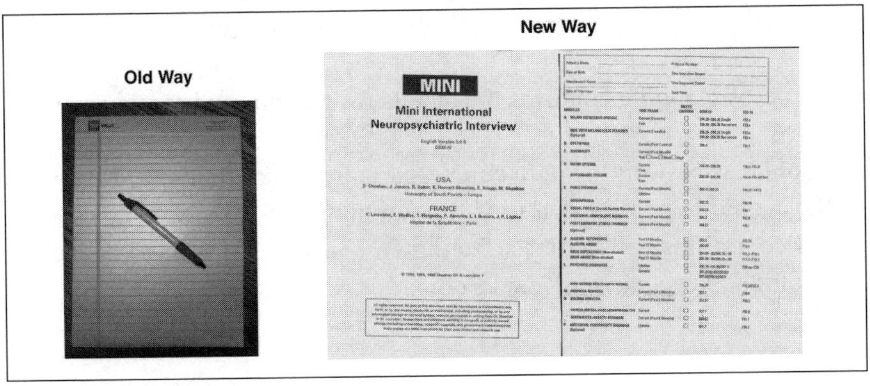

Figure 6-13. Standardized work: Making sure consistent information is taken from every patient during the initial contact is important to making best use of the office visit. Standardizing information with an agreed-upon form has saved time and rework.

"The tool made it easier," said Sobota, "but once the nurses all got trained, they began making more refinements to it. Conducting the evaluations ahead of time by phone just increases the nurses' value as 'physician extenders' and reduces how long patients have to wait in the office."

Six evaluations can now be completed in the time it took to do four. Overtime has decreased. The time patients spend waiting for the doctor is down 17 percent, the time they spend with the doctor is up by 7 percent, and their time with the nurse is up 10 percent. (Figures 6-14, 6-15)

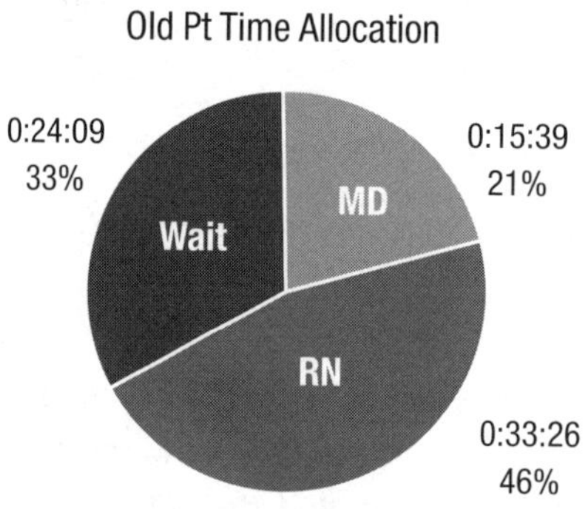

Figure 6-14. Time allocation before improvements.

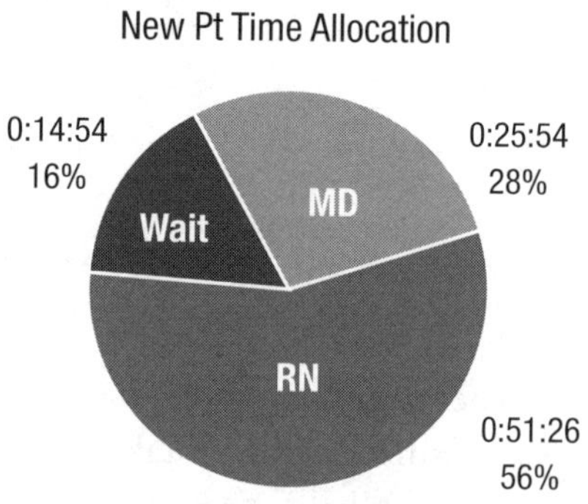

Figure 6-15. Time allocation after improvements. Patients spend 17 percent less time waiting, 10 percent more time with nurses, and 7 percent more time with doctors.

Process mapping confirms the results for patients and caregivers (Figure 6-16).

Sobota is networking with counterparts from the Children's Hospital's CDU, in an effort to shorten waits for appointments.

"I've got this new tool, Perfecting Patient Care. It's like a stick, and I'm going to keep stirring," said Sobota.

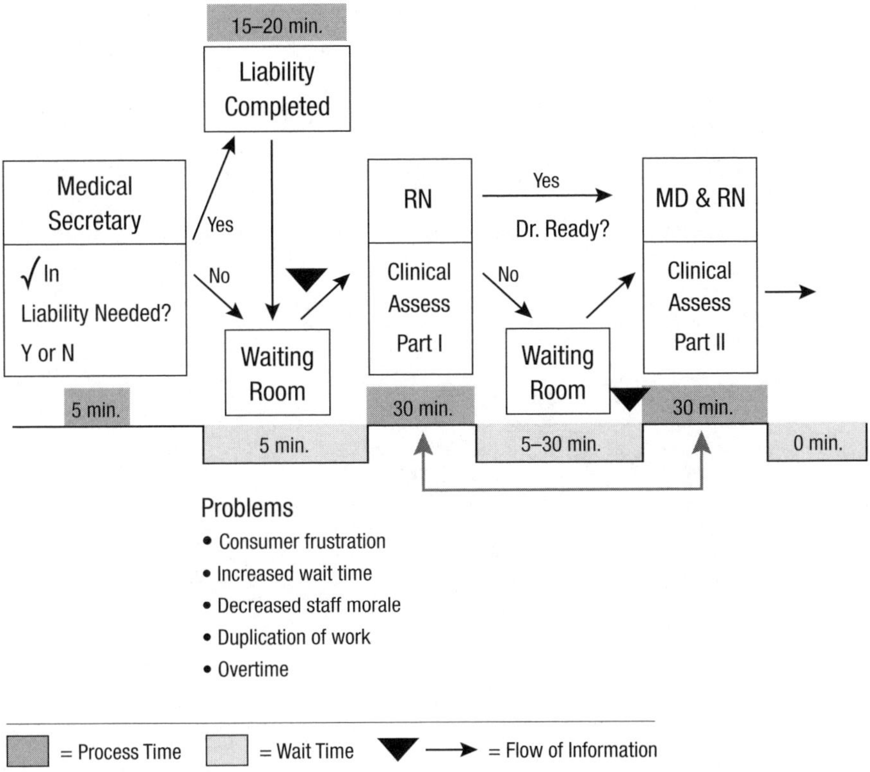

Figure 6-16. Revisiting the process map after experiments confirm whether or not improvement has actually taken place. With wait time significantly decreased, the patient leaves the encounter happy.

CHAPTER 7

Applying Best Practices

CASE STUDIES

- **Section 1. Can controlling blood glucose reduce postsurgical infections?** Veterans Administration Pittsburgh Healthcare System (VAPHS) physician, Harsha Rao, MD presented a glucose control protocol to the community that is being used for tight control of blood glucose following cardiac surgery. The result is declining infection rates.
- **Section 2. Best diabetes care applied in two community health centers.** The advantages of the renowned Wagner Model for delivering diabetes care are beyond dispute. Actually implementing the Wagner Model is difficult. Eileen Boyle, MD, a physician with a local, federally qualified health center, finds that Perfecting Patient Care makes the Wagner Model easier to use.
- **Section 3. Building a better diabetes appointment.** Instead of the patient going to a series of doctors, Harsha Rao, MD, and the team of healthcare providers at the VAPHS surround each patient during a one-hour appointment.
- **Section 4. Nine myths about electronic medical records.** While electronic fixes may not always pan out, one private practice decided to take a bold leap, installing an expensive electronic medical record system without delay. The results have paid off for patients, physicians, and healthcare professionals alike.

When a large cross-section of a staff has a basic understanding of the principles of Perfecting Patient Care, the ensuing work redesign seems to result in less waste and better quality of care. These improvements seem to take hold regardless of the healthcare organization in which the techniques are applied—hospitals (large or small), community clinics, or private physicians' offices. Because so many of the case studies in this book describe work in hospitals, it is important to note that the principles of work redesign have also been applied to medical care that seems resistant to improvement, namely, chronic care.

Chronic illnesses like diabetes, asthma, and congestive heart failure affect more than 90 million people in the United States and account for 75 percent of the nation's healthcare outlays, according to the CDC, which estimates that diabetes alone costs more than $132 billion.

Care of chronic illness is often marked by expense, waste, inefficiencies, and variations in practice and outcomes. For example, one in seven hospital admissions occur because care providers do not have access to previous medical records. And 20 percent of lab tests are requested because previous results are not accessible.

American healthcare is structured to care for acute diseases. But chronic diseases like diabetes require a different kind of care: sustained, coordinated medical service along with patient education. The current medical system is not set up financially or systemically to do that very well. The result: a landmark 2003 RAND study[1] revealed that on average, Americans receive recommended care for chronic illnesses only 55 percent of the time. Among diabetic patients, it's just 45 percent.

Failure to deliver consistently adequate care for chronic disease leads to serious—and largely preventable—complications. Among diabetics, these include blindness, renal failure, and heart disease.

Financial incentives misaligned

Care for patients with chronic diseases, like diabetes, provides an instructive example of the perverse incentives inherent in the current system. To deliver comprehensive diabetes care, a number of routine tests are required—from glucose and blood pressure management, to blood tests measuring hemoglobin A1C[2] and lipid levels,[3] to foot and eye exams. Physicians find it impossible to do everything in one poorly reimbursed

1. Elizabeth A. McGlynn, PhD, et al., "The Quality of Health Care Delivered to Adults in the United States," *N Engl J Med* 348:26, 2635–2645 (June 26, 2003).

eight-minute office visit. Often, physicians are not paid for multiple tests performed during a single office visit. Diabetic patients, unable to keep up with a blizzard of appointments, are unlikely to receive the consistent care they need. The result is an explosion of preventable, life-threatening complications, such as blindness, amputation, and kidney failure, all of which are devastating to patients and exponentially more expensive to treat than diabetes itself.

Many insurers are exploring alternative payment structures, like "pay for performance," as a way to reward efficiency. They are realizing that incentives are not aligned to encourage the most effective treatments. Currently processes, not outcomes, are rewarded: Consensus is slowly building that that equation needs to be reversed.

Federal programs less constrained

Federal health insurance, which includes the Veterans Administration Health Care System (VA) and Federally Qualified Health Centers (FQHCs), cover about a quarter of all Americans with health insurance.[4] The VA and FQHCs are "closed" systems, where clinicians are employees, and the compensation system does not penalize improved efficiency.

Improvements to diabetes care in federally funded systems could provide important "proof of concept" for Perfecting Patient Care. That's why PRHI has engaged in demonstration projects aimed at improving care for diabetic patients: one at the VA Pittsburgh Healthcare System (VAPHS) under Dr. Harsha Rao; one at the FQHC in Lawrenceville with Jan Setzenfand, RN; and one at the FQHC in East Liberty under Dr. Eileen Boyle.

---

2. A blood test that shows the average amount of glucose in the blood over the past three months. The result indicates whether the blood sugar level is under control, which is important in the management of diabetes.
3. More commonly known as cholesterol levels.
4. Executive Order: Promoting Quality and Efficient Health Care in Federal Government Administered or Sponsored Health Care Programs, Washington, D.C., August 2006.

• SECTION 1 •

CAN CONTROLLING BLOOD GLUCOSE REDUCE POSTSURGICAL INFECTIONS?

Harsha Rao, MD, Professsor of Medicine and Chief of Endocrinology at the VAPHS, believes in tight control of insulin in postoperative cardiac surgery patients. Why? Research shows that tight blood glucose control helps eliminate postsurgical infections, especially the devastating, deep sternal wound infection known as mediastinitis.[5] Clinicians in the surgical intensive care unit (SICU) at the VAPHS have tested a dynamic, easy-to-use program to administer the exacting postsurgical insulin protocol with encouraging results.

Dr. Rao outlines the problem this way: For decades, a single formula, or sliding scale, has been used to determine the insulin drip rate for every patient in every situation in an attempt to achieve the target blood glucose (BG) level of between 80–110. The simple, one-size-fits-all formula takes the current BG number, minus 80, times 0.03–.05.

---

5. S. S. Kowli, "Insulin and sepsis," *J Postgrad Med* 31:11–5 (1985).
It has recently been recognized that hyperglycemia is a significant risk factor for postoperative infectious complications. Hyperglycemia in the postoperative patient occurs on the basis of postoperative insulin resistance, a transient state of reduced sensitivity to the anabolic effects of insulin. This state, similar to Type 2 diabetes mellitus, is not traditionally treated in routine perioperative care. Development of methods to attenuate postoperative insulin resistance may improve outcome of surgical care.

Mattias Soop, *Effects of perioperative nutrition on insulin action in postoperative metabolism*. Fredagen den 16 maj 2003, kl. 9.00, Ersta Sköndals aula, Stigbergsgatan 30, Stockholm.

The majority of hospitalizations for patients with diabetes are due to comorbid conditions, and diabetes management is not a focus during inpatient stays. However, inpatient hyperglycemia has been associated with nosocomial infections, increased mortality and increased length of stay.

D. Baldwin, *Diabetes Care* 28:1008–1011 (2005).

Sliding scale limitations

"This formula is completely empirical, based on a regression line drawn years ago. The target is rarely, if ever, achieved," said Dr. Rao, "because it doesn't take into account changes in the glucose reading over time." Table 7-1 shows an example of the formula's shortcomings: Each patient in the example has had different spikes in prior BG readings and should receive different doses of insulin, yet the formula dictates the same amount.

Table 7–1. Time-honored "Sliding Scale" Formula has Shortcomings

Time-honored "Sliding Scale" Formula has Shortcomings	
It does not take into account blood glucose readings over time. Examples:	
BG 150 each of past 2 hours	Drip rate: $(150\text{-}80) \times 0.03 = 2.1$u/hr.
BG 150 now, was 240 last hour	Drip rate: $(150\text{-}80) \times 0.03 = 2.1$u/hr.
BG 150 now, was 100 last hour	Drip rate: $(150\text{-}80) \times 0.03 = 2.1$u/hr.

Dr. Rao asked, "This formula applies to every patient, but in reality does it apply to even one?"

Complex formula—easy to use

Peter Perreiah, PRHI's managing director, developed an Excel-based user interface that enables a nurse to use a sophisticated algorithm developed by Dr. Rao and his team at the VAPHS to determine exactly how much insulin each patient needs at any given time. This "wizard" allows constant, precise alteration of the insulin drip to enable tight BG control.

The goals of the VAPHS' insulin protocol are to:

1. Prevent hypoglycemia (low blood sugar). Although clinically, hyperglycemia (high blood sugar) is a far bigger threat to patients' health, nurses' training generally leads to a bigger fear of hypoglycemia. The emphasis on preventing hypoglycemia is a way to overcome nurses' discomfort, addressing a cultural barrier in a clinical way.

2. Bring BG into the 80–110 mg/dL range within four hours of protocol use.
3. Maintain glucose in the 80–110 mg/dL range, avoiding swings in BG often seen in patients in the intensive care unit.

The wizard then displays the recommended drip rate, when to check again, and any other alerts.

Heeding the voice of the nurse

The nurses, who are responsible for implementing the protocol, give constant feedback about the utility of the software and how to improve it based on floor use. The VAPHS is on the 17th version of the software, with ever-improving results. Of the 93 patients placed on the protocol postsurgically, only one developed an infection—traced to a deviation in the protocol.

Candace Cunningham, RN, SICU team leader notes, "In the beginning, the nurses thought that constant attention to the protocol would be frustrating. Now, they are frustrated when they can't get the patient's blood glucose to stay in the target range. The protocol lets them concentrate on the patient."

Cunningham adds, "When we say we want blood glucose between 80 and 110, we mean 80 to 110. Before, we would have felt good about 150; now that's unacceptable."

Problems arose when, once BG readings were within the target range, physicians would stop the insulin drip, assuming the hyperglycemia to be resolved. However, BG readings often rose again and began fluctuating wildly once the insulin was stopped. Now, termination of the drip protocol is not left to the physician, unless the patient has uncontrolled hyper- or hypoglycemia.

Step-down challenges

When a patient moves to the step-down unit, a transitional insulin protocol is needed that takes into account the increased patient–nurse ratio. (In the SICU, the ratio is one-to-one for the first 12 hours, then two patients per nurse thereafter until transfer to the step-down unit, where the ratio is four patients to one nurse). When a patient in the step-down unit begins to eat, monitoring insulin levels can become more complicated. Actually, food consumption posed two new considerations:

1. The postoperative cardiac diet specified no caffeine or salt, but did not specify the carbohydrate count. Once alerted, the VAPHS dieticians quickly ensured a standardized carbohydrate count for each cardiac post-op tray.
2. Busy nurses needed to assess how much each patient consumed after each meal so that they could administer insulin after meal consumption. Giving insulin after the meal allows them to base the dose on a straightforward formula per 15 grams of carbohydrates consumed.

"I was delighted to realize that asking nurses to estimate food consumption did not add to their workloads," said Dr. Rao. "They are already trained from nursing school to assess how much the patient has eaten." Now that bit of data, which they already collect, increases in importance.

Again, the dynamic transitional protocol is capable of sophisticated calculations needed to meet each patient's need and is easy to use. The result shows exactly how much insulin and in what form to administer it, as well as other necessary information. Like the SICU protocol, the transitional protocol is under continuous development and improvement.

New frontiers

The next frontier in glucose control is further upstream, in the operating room (OR). There, another version of the insulin protocol software is being developed and refined. The hope is that preventing swings in patients' BG levels from the start of surgery may further help reduce post-surgical infections.

The patient then combats the final frontier by bringing home the concept of tight glycemic control when he or she discharges from the hospital. The wound is only partially healed when this happens, so that the potential for complications is still very real, particularly because patients often have little or no support for aggressive diabetes management at a time when they are struggling to adapt to postoperative life outside the hospital following such a major surgical procedure. Conquering this problem will require a different approach, involving the provision of adequate resources to enable far more frequent contact between the diabetes care team and the patient.

Despite vigorous attempts to control the bacterial 'seed' of infection by asepsis and antibiotics, infection is still the greatest enemy of surgeons. Hence, more attention is now being focused on the 'soil' or host factors and their contribution to postoperative infection. Numerous works have confirmed hyperglycemia as a metabolic response to operative stress. Inquiry and improvement continue.

• SECTION 2 •

BEST DIABETES CARE APPLIED IN TWO COMMUNITY HEALTH CENTERS

Like federally qualified health centers nationwide, the UPMC St. Margaret Lawrenceville Family Health Clinic (LFHC) is implementing the Wagner Model of Chronic Care, which originated with Dr. Ed Wagner at Seattle's MacColl Institute for Healthcare Innovation. The Wagner Chronic Care Model is generally believed the standard of care for people with diabetes and other chronic illnesses. Since such a model exists, shouldn't it be easy to make sure every diabetic person receives the treatment outlined in the Wagner Model?

What is the Wagner Model?

The Chronic Care Model identifies the essential elements of a healthcare system that encourage high-quality chronic disease care. These elements, each representing a significant content area, are:

- The community,
- The health system,
- Self-management support,
- Delivery system design,
- Decision support, and
- Clinical information systems.

The model was created by Ed H. Wagner, MD, MH, FACP, director of Improving Chronic Illness Care (ICIC), a general internist/epidemiologist, and director of the Seattle-based MacColl Institute for Healthcare Innovation. He has developed and tested population-based care models for diabetes, frailty in the elderly and other chronic illnesses; the evaluation of the health and cost impacts of health promotion/disease prevention interventions; and interventions to prevent disability and reduce depressive symptoms in older adults. He has written two books and more than 200 publications.

Additional information is available at http://www.centerforhealthstudies.org/research/maccoll.html.

The best care will not help people who do not come in to receive it. When workers at the UPMC St. Margaret LFHC decided to apply the principles of Perfecting Patient Care to their work with diabetic patients, they immediately ran into problems. Just finding all of the diabetic patients required a tedious, time-consuming chart review.

The staff at LFHC used a one-at-a-time approach to create a database of all diabetic patients. They follow up with doctors and staff to ensure that anyone newly diagnosed, or any new patient with diabetes, is added to the list. They follow lab results to see who is getting regular blood tests, eye exams, and so forth, and cross check with reports from insurance agencies. They identify people with barriers to care. Now:

- Patients who may have missed a blood test or a checkup receive a reminder letter or even a phone call. As a result, regular, scheduled visits by diabetic patients are way up.
- Every month, 30 to 40 patients are invited to class to learn ways to manage their diabetes. As attendance has picked up, 60 percent of patients are coming to class, and 95 percent of attendees have shown clinical improvement.

In Southwestern Pennsylvania: What We Know and Why it Matters

Improperly managed diabetes is a leading cause of blindness, limb amputation, cardiovascular disease, and kidney failure. Nationwide, deaths from diabetes have risen 58 percent since 1979. Five counties in Southwestern Pennsylvania, (Beaver, Butler, Fayette, Washington, and Westmoreland) all report higher rates of complications and death from diabetes than the state average.* Diabetes hits particularly hard among Southwestern Pennsylvania's African Americans, who, for example, undergo twice as many limb amputations as whites.

Patients with diabetes receive routine care—eye and foot exams, kidney monitoring, lipid screening and control—between 9 percent and 57 percent of the time. In other words, despite the best efforts of our medical professionals, only about half of known diabetics receive appropriate treatment.

The region saw a shocking 75 percent increase in hospitalizations due to diabetic complications between 1997 and 2001 at a cost of $1.27 billion in hospital charges.

The suffering is made all the more unacceptable, because diabetic complications leading to hospitalization are almost always preventable.

**Results of a special study conducted for PRHI by the Pennsylvania Health Care Cost Containment Council, 2001.*

Of the 13,000 patients seen at LFHC, about 260 are known to have diabetes. Making sure that all of those patients receive recommended care at each visit, plus the education they need to manage their condition, has become a cause for team leader Jan Setzenfand, RN. Jan took the Perfecting Patient Care University, with the idea of applying the improvement techniques specifically to the care of diabetic patients. On-site coaching was provided by PRHI teacher, Fran Sheedy-Bost.

"This is where the Wagner Model and Perfecting Patient Care meet. The model tells us what care a diabetic patient needs: Perfecting Patient Care gives us practical ways we can make sure it happens," says Setzenfand.

Beginning with a question

Perfecting Patient Care often begins with one simple question. In this case, the team considered: Do our exam rooms make it possible to deliver perfect care to diabetic patients every time?

Trained observers noticed physicians and nurses leaving exam rooms repeatedly during patient encounters to find items that were not in the room, robbing precious minutes from the exam. Setzenfand's team discovered that no two exam rooms were equipped quite alike. For example, none had large blood-pressure cuffs for heavier patients, since they were stored in a separate room. None contained a monofilament, a pen-sized instrument for measuring foot sensation, which is required every time a diabetic patient comes in for care (Figures 7-1 and 7-2).

Drawing on what they had learned from visiting the Perfecting Patient Care team at the VAPHS, and collaborating with the entire staff, Setzenfand's group set about creating a "perfect"

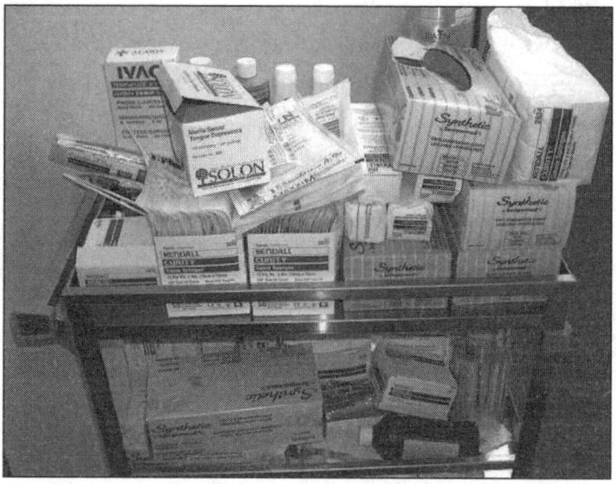

Figure 7-1. Hundreds of dollars in unused inventory came out of exam rooms.

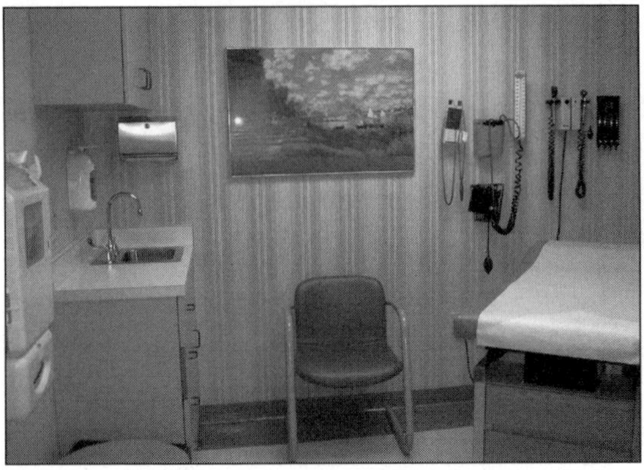

Figure 7-2. What remained was *only* and *all* of what was needed for routine exams. Each exam room is now arranged and stocked identically.

exam room—one with the right items in the right amounts for examining diabetic patients. Counters were cleared to increase workspace (Figures 7-3 and 7-4). Soon staff members were adjusting the room to ensure the right items were there for every usual need. In all, they made 15 improvements.

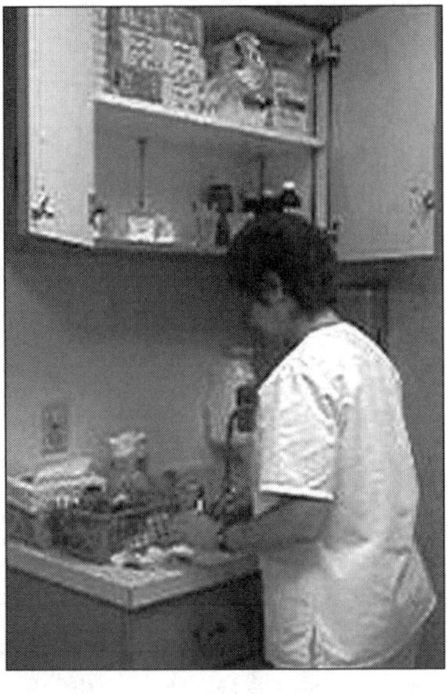

Figure 7-3. *Before:* Cluttered workspace wasted clinician time.

The staff quickly developed a preference for using the "perfect" exam room for all patients, not just those with diabetes. So the team standardized every room into a perfect room: unused inventory came out and needed supplies—like large blood-pressure cuffs and monofilaments—went in.

Physicians can now do more for patients during office visits. The standardized rooms made orientation for new clinicians much easier. Improvements made ostensibly, in the interest of diabetic patients, began to accrue to all patients.

"This isn't just about cleaning out rooms. It's about getting people exactly what they need, when they need it. Improving work flow definitely relates to clinical improvements," says Setzenfand.

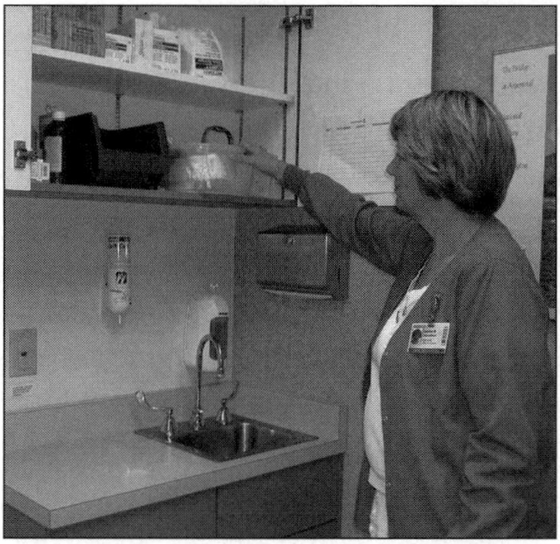

Figure 7-4. *After:* Organized supplies mean more workspace, plus time for clinician to spend on direct patient care. Workers have *all* they need and *only* what they need.

Visual cues

Perfecting Patient Care techniques often rely on visual cues. From posters to Post-Its®, visual reminders either inform or reinforce desired practice and help people do the right thing. Visual cues can help clinicians, patients, and even suppliers of goods and services, like outside laboratories.

For example, diabetic patients require foot exams at each visit. Setzenfand and team discovered, as they went chart by chart, variation in the frequency and documentation of foot exams. Working with the physicians, the team devised a simple sticker for each chart that provided: 1) a reminder to do the exam, and 2) a consistent way to chart what had been done.

Diabetic patients also require a yearly, dilated eye exam to check for retinal damage. Since blindness is such a devastating potential complication for diabetics, annual eye exams are extremely important. But many of the center's patients misunderstood or overlooked verbal instructions to have their eyes tested. So the team devised a prescription-like pad describing the needed test, including the reason, the frequency, and the physician phone numbers. Physicians and patients found the pads easy to use. Of the patients who received the form, 93 percent presented themselves for a dilated eye exam.

Lab tests posed another challenge. An internal form listed all the tests necessary for diabetics, but the commercial lab's form was different and hard to use. As a result of a meeting between the center's medical director and a lab representative, the forms were standardized, and the lab amended its form.

Diabetes registry

The best care will not help people who do not come in to receive it. The staff at LFHC used a one-at-a-time approach to create a registry of patients, identifying people with barriers to care, and taking steps to help them reach optimal health. They created a database of all diabetic patients, and followed up with doctors and staff members to ensure that anyone newly diagnosed, or any new patient with diabetes, is added to the list. They also follow lab results to see who is getting regular blood tests, eye exams, and so forth, and they cross check this information with reports from insurance agencies. Benefits include:

- Those patients who may have missed a blood test or a checkup receive a reminder letter or even a phone call. Regular, scheduled visits by diabetic patients are up.
- Every month, 30 to 40 patients are invited to class to learn ways to manage their diabetes. As attendance has picked up, 60 percent of patients are coming to class, and 95 percent of attendees have shown clinical improvement (Figure 7-5).

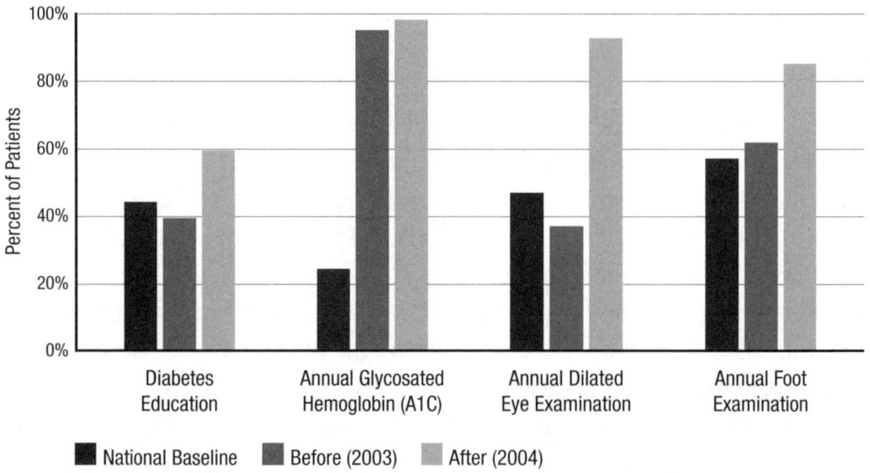

Figure 7-5. Application of Perfecting Patient Care Has Improved Outcomes at the Lawerenceville Family Health Center.

APPLYING THE WAGNER MODEL USING PERFECTING PATIENT CARE

As part of her Physician Champion grant, Eileen Boyle, MD, is overseeing implementation of the Wagner Chronic Care Model with diabetic patients and others with chronic illnesses at East Liberty Family Health Center, another Pittsburgh-area, federally qualified health center (FQHC). In a recently aired PBS documentary on chronic care,[6] Dr. Wagner said, "Those who stand the best chance of receiving comprehensive chronic care are those relying on the public health system." He cited the lack of properly reimbursed preventive care among private insurance plans.

Dr. Boyle believes all medical practices will need new approaches to chronic care as private insurers and Medicare begin to pay for performance, emphasizing outcomes over the number of episodes of care a patient receives. But for now, her goal remains implementing and spreading the Wagner Model at East Liberty's two sites where she provides chronic care.

Training brings results

Through the Physician Champion Program, Dr. Boyle and team are learning how to apply Perfecting Patient Care in their workplace and receiving coaching from PRHI's Learning Center Director, Mimi Falbo, MSN. Falbo, along with Barbara Jennion, MA, and Tania Lyon, PhD, have spent the past two years upgrading and improving the Perfecting Patient Care curriculum for the Nurse Navigators and Physician Champions. Dr. Boyle says that the resulting work redesign is already producing improvements.

For example, a cornerstone of the Chronic Care Model calls for patients to set their own goals for improving their care. When Dr. Boyle's team measured patient goal setting for the first time, "We started out at 1 percent," she said. "The self management goal setting was either not being done or not being documented, but with the last report, after examining and improving processes using Perfecting Patient Care, we were up to 72 percent."

---

6. "Remaking American Medicine," PBS, Frank Christopher and Matt Eisan, filmmakers.

Wrong kinds of appointments

Recent improvements to the clinic's scheduling process have increased patient and caregiver satisfaction while reducing the number of "no shows."

Falbo says "The team mapped the entire path of a patient going through their system (Figure 7-6). Once they saw the whole patient encounter, they quickly zeroed in on scheduling as a prime problem. Why was the doctor so often called out of the room during a patient visit? Frequently it was to see whether that doctor could squeeze in just one more patient."

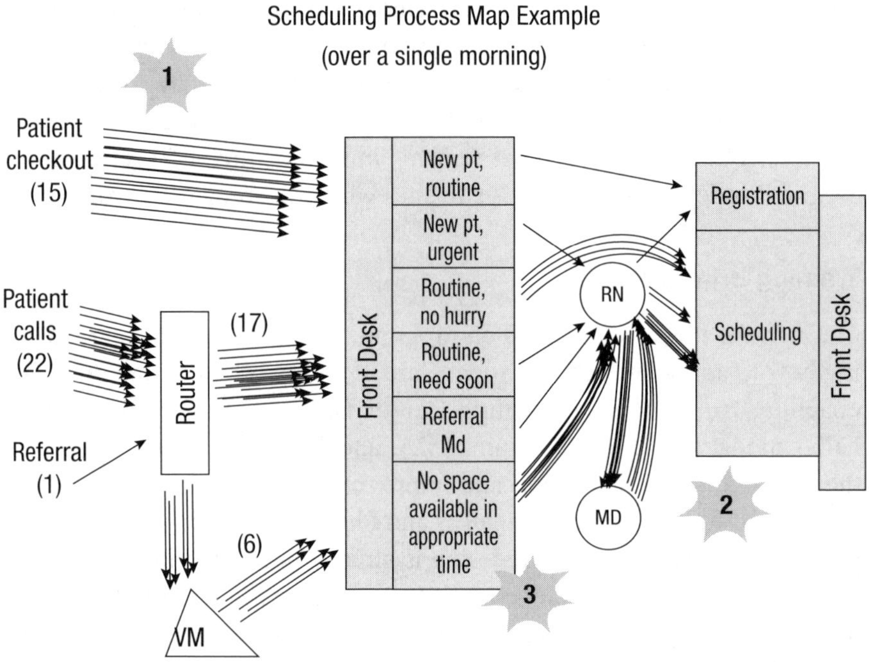

Figure 7-6. Process mapping helps clarify opportunities for improvement. The jagged symbols around areas 1, 2, and 3 indicate areas where problems need to be examined further.

Asking a series of "Why" questions led the team to discover the glitch: the way appointments were scheduled. Related problems surfaced, such as large fluctuations in the workload. The clinic could be crushed with activity, or idle when patients failed to keep appointments. "No shows" were a special concern regarding diabetic patients, who must be seen at regular intervals.

"We were overproducing the wrong kinds of appointments," said Falbo.

Preparing for open access

Together, the entire team committed to the ambitious goal of creating "open access" time in the schedule. This would enable them to set an appointment within 24 hours of the patient's phone call, with that patient's primary care physician (PCP). It wasn't easy. Because some patients had habitually seen the first available doctor, they had to be assigned a PCP.

Other logistics required advanced planning. The team had to agree on how much open time to leave in the schedule, and when. They realized that, once the system came online, rapid-cycle improvements might require further change.

Office staff members created and standardized their own system of callbacks for diabetic patients. Now, if a patient fails to call for a regular appointment, that patient will receive a call or postcard from an office staffer to arrange the appointment.

To prepare patients for the new "open access" appointments, office staff created a blue flyer describing the changes and handed them out to each patient for several weeks before the changeover.

Members of the entire care team met to write scripts for the telephone staff. The scripts covered basic information about the new appointment system, but included a detailed flow chart covering frequently asked questions. A beneficial side effect of the scripting is that telephone staff now also have a better idea of when to involve a nurse or a doctor with a patient question.

Success from the start

On October 1, 2006 after two months of planning, the clinic switched over to open access scheduling with nary a glitch. Progress charts hang proudly in employee areas of each clinic, comparing before and after rates of no-shows, percentage of time patients get to see their own PCPs, and other quality measures. Even the measures are organized. Staff decides what they will measure and who will track and measure it this month. The work is evenly distributed and everyone agrees on what is being measured.

"Implementing Perfecting Patient Care has helped us design and standardize the work," said Dr. Boyle. "The successful changeover of our appointment system has generated a lot of excitement on the staff. There's no more 'dead time' followed by 'crush time.' Staff feels like they have more control over their environment, and more freedom to do a better job."

Doctors and nurses, now able to have time to give more complete care, do their charting, and create the systems they need to implement the Chronic Care Model. From a modest two doctors and 17 diabetic patients in one clinic, the Chronic Care Model now covers three doctors and 207 diabetic patients in two clinics. The goal is to have all providers using the program, covering all 500+ diabetics.

Results

Since the experiments began, a diabetic patient due for an appointment can get one within a day. No-shows have decreased from 40 percent to 15 percent. In just the first four weeks, productivity improved to 1.7 patients per hour, up from 1.3.

"A new issue is empty slots—of which we had none before," said Dr. Boyle. The empty slots were among pediatric physicians, so the group is calling families whose children are due for well child care.

"We clearly see that Perfecting Patient Care techniques offer an organized way to spread the Chronic Care Model," says Dr. Boyle.

• SECTION 3 •

BUILDING A BETTER DIABETES APPOINTMENT

Dr. Harsha Rao is changing his clinic's approach to treating diabetes to a team model. Doing so, he believes, will not only enable him to provide more comprehensive care and improve outcomes, but allow him to see more patients. An endocrinologist at the VA Pittsburgh Health System (VAPHS), Dr. Rao has been working with PRHI to implement the new model with assistance from the Physician Champion program.

Comprehensive diabetes care

In comprehensive diabetes care, inefficiency remains a problem for both patients and physicians because of the number of routine interventions and tests required—from glucose and blood pressure management, to blood tests measuring hemoglobin A1C and lipid levels, to foot and eye exams. Physicians find it nearly impossible to do everything in a single visit, and patients often can't afford the time for multiple appointments. The setup makes suboptimal care and outcomes almost inevitable.

Increasing the big three: intensity, volume, and personalized care

Dr. Rao had been thinking about the team approach to diabetes care—and refining it in theory—over the past 25 years. With the help of PRHI, he is now implementing it and testing its effectiveness in practice. He believes his new approach blends the best of the group model that is slowly gaining acceptance across the United States, with the individual patient visits that have long been the norm.

The group model "gives you volume without personalized care and intensity," he said, while the typical individual patient visit in the United States "gives you the intensity of one-on-one attention without the volume."

Dr. Rao said his team approach "combines intensity, volume, and personalized care." It also can fill in gaps in care, such as nutrition and diabetes education, that many physicians are not trained to deliver, yet are proven to help patients manage their disease better.

A role for each team member

Along with Dr. Rao, the Pittsburgh VA team consists of a nurse educator, a pharmacist, a nutritionist, and a nurse practitioner. The patient spends roughly 15 minutes at each "station." Dr. Rao "floats" between all stations, observing and troubleshooting as necessary. Tania Lyon, PhD, assistant director of PRHI's chronic-care initiative and coordinator of the Physician Champions program, is the coach at Dr. Rao's clinic.

As a physician, Dr. Rao's role is limited to those tasks that he was trained to pursue, such as glucose, blood pressure, and cholesterol management. Those goals remain unchanged in the new team model. But the team model aims to improve efficiency by allowing multiple practitioners to perform all necessary tasks for each patient in a single, hour-long session. Each patient's encounter becomes a comprehensive-care experience.

In fact, as soon as he adds ophthalmologic care, as he plans to do in the near future, each patient visit will amount to "one-stop shopping," Dr. Rao said.

Increased efficiency = increased volume

Once the new model becomes routine, Dr. Rao predicts his team members will be able to deliver comprehensive care to four patients every hour. As a result, he projects the clinic's volume will expand to 16 patients during its four-hour sessions.

He is phasing in the changes to ensure that patient care does not suffer while team members acclimate to the routine. Like all Physician Champion participants, Dr. Rao will document and measure outcomes as he proceeds.

A reimbursement system in the way

No matter how successful the experiment, however, don't expect widespread adoption of Dr. Rao's team model any time soon.

"The difficulty of implementing such a model in the private sector is that insurance companies don't reimburse for more than one professional visit for the same diagnosis on the same day," Dr. Rao said. In fact, some of the routine services that his team provides, such as nutrition counseling and diabetes education, often are not reimbursed under private health plans, even when they're provided during separate visits.

The VA Health System's federal funding and salaried staff make the team approach financially feasible. For practitioners who must bill private health plans or Medicare, it may not be.

Industrial concept works

Setting up a system in which different clinicians do different tasks associated with a patient's care is somewhat akin to setting up a production line, Dr. Rao said. He said PRHI's coaching in Perfecting Patient Care principles helped with the implementation of his model. Dr. Rao said the methods were directly responsible for the fact that the team increased the flow of patients during its 4-hour afternoon sessions from 8 to 12 on just the third attempt (Figure 7-7).

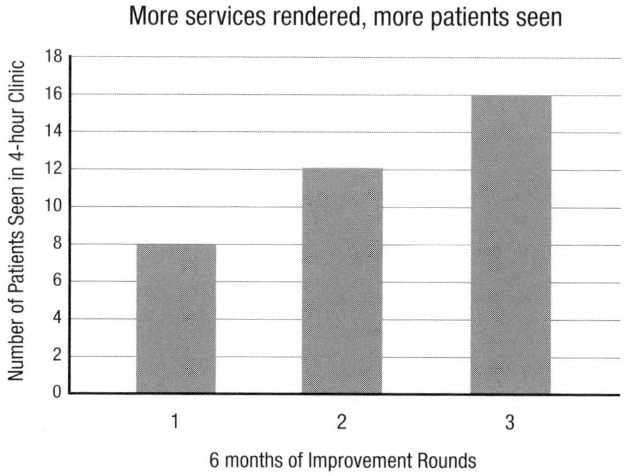

Figure 7-7. In Just Three Tries, 1/3 More Patients Seen and Better Care Rendered.

Importance of training

"The facts that we attended formal training in these techniques and have had Dr. Tania Lyon, an outside observer, has helped us make better choices and to improve the model as we've gone along" said Dr. Rao. "Tania points out things that we do not see, and we sit down (as soon as a problem arises) to have a discussion about how to fix it."

• SECTION 4 •

NINE MYTHS ABOUT ELECTRONIC MEDICAL RECORDS

That it will ever come into general use notwithstanding its value is extremely doubtful; because its beneficial application requires much time and gives a good bit of trouble both to the patient and the practitioner; because its hue and character are foreign, and opposed to all our habits and associations.

—London Times, *1834, in reaction to Laennec's introduction of the stethoscope*

Paper and the unassisted mind are no longer sufficient for today's standard of care. As former House Speaker Newt Gingrich said, "Paper kills." Gingrich founded the Center for Health Transformation, a public/ private partnership urging technological reforms in healthcare.

An electronic medical record (EMR) is seen as the fulcrum on which high-quality, efficient chronic care rests. The staff at the UPMC St. Margaret Lawrenceville Family Health Clinic (LFHC) created their own simple registry, focused strictly on providing high-quality care for patients, one at a time.

Currently, most electronic systems focus on improving the efficiency and accuracy of scheduling and billing. Few have designed their software with a model of care in mind. Software components that assist clinical performance, when they are developed at all, are added on as afterthoughts.

Physicians need an electronic system that can help them identify, for example, which diabetic patients have not come in for a follow-up visit in the recommended 3- to 6-month period, or which ones need dilated retinal exams. Most EMRs have individual patient-record templates that would allow this, but lack a registry function that would allow doctors to track overall performance.

Physicians need electronic systems that allow them to trend their own evidence-based care over time—to pinpoint areas for improvement. For example, what percentage of diabetic patients received dilated, retinal eye exams last year, or monofilament foot exams with each visit?

With paper systems, such as LFHC's, gathering basic data requires hours of intensive chart review. With the right electronic system, these data could be regularly incorporated, revolutionizing the way care is delivered and improved upon.

To make the most of an EMR, therefore, it is not enough to simply "plug and play"—overlay a digital system over the current method of doing work. The power for EMRs to affect quality lies in their ability to illuminate work processes and help redesign them.

Who pays? Who benefits?

The United States lags behind other Western countries in adopting a national standard for electronic medical records. In the United States, large hospital systems are more likely to have capital to invest in a conversion to EMRs than small, solo physician practices.

But while most Americans get their healthcare from small practices, only 15 percent of all primary care physicians and 6 percent of solo practitioners have EMRs.

In spite of a growing interest, EMRs cost about $10,000 to $30,000 per physician—a daunting barrier to practices operating on slim profit margins. An additional barrier is the misaligned incentive. Although primary care practices hold the key to digitizing patients' records—especially the chronically ill—only about 11 percent of the captured savings are likely to accrue to the investing physician.

The reason: Reimbursement systems rarely reward increased efficiency.

Private practitioner won't wait to innovate

Innovations in healthcare have historically been met with skepticism. Studies confirm that it takes an average of 17 years for valid medical practices to move from publication to adoption in the field. The electronic medical record (EMR) is an innovation that holds transformative possibilities for physician practices.

- One out of every seven hospital admissions occurs because clinicians don't have access to previous medical records, and 20 percent of lab tests are requested because previous results have

been lost. EMRs ensure that patients' records can be easily retrieved, reducing the chances of duplicate testing and medication interactions.
- Recent studies estimate that close to 30 percent of medical errors result from a lack of available information at the time a decision is made.
- Currently, people with diabetes and other chronic illnesses receive "best practice" care less than half of the time. With sophisticated decision-support capabilities, EMR software can increase the chances that best practices will be applied.
- In terms of reimbursement, EMR software streamlines coding and billing and reduces the strain on office staff.

Even with these powerful incentives, EMR adoption in private practices is catching on slowly—too slowly for Dr. William Fera, a Pittsburgh-area general practitioner. He and his partner, Dr. Joel Diamond, along with others in their group, decided to invest in an EMR even though it was expensive (about $80,000 per year), and no other entity would help them pay for it.

Today, Dr. Fera is an EMR evangelist, telling as many physicians as will listen about the efficiencies his practice has gained in the four years since its installation. A self-styled mythbuster, Dr. Fera addresses the top nine reasons physicians give for not purchasing an EMR system.

1. It costs too much.

   "People tend to ask about money first," says Dr. Fera. "But EMRs are important because they reduce wasted time and improve quality. In the end, EMRs allow you to improve patient care while actually saving/making money. That is the real irony here."

   Using his practice as an example, Dr. Fera says reduced baseline expenses fell into three categories: the lease on the existing billing/data system; 2.5 FTEs from support staff; and transcription service. Those services totaled nearly $175,000 per year. The lease on the new EMR cost about $80,000. All told, he saved over $94,000 in the first year.

   The savings only compounded in the second year. The costs for charting and dictation simply evaporated; coding improved (Figure 7-8); overtime was greatly reduced. In fact, the practice was able to run more efficiently with four fewer employees. (This efficiency relied on natural attrition, not layoffs. Workers must understand that innovations will not cost them their jobs.) Productivity is up, claim denials are down, and turnaround time for reimbursement is faster.

Getting beyond the "hard cost" of the EMR system, other efficiencies are gained by improving the quality of care. With access to each patient's data, and to clinical guidelines and reporting software, every practice can benchmark itself against best practices and continuously improve care.

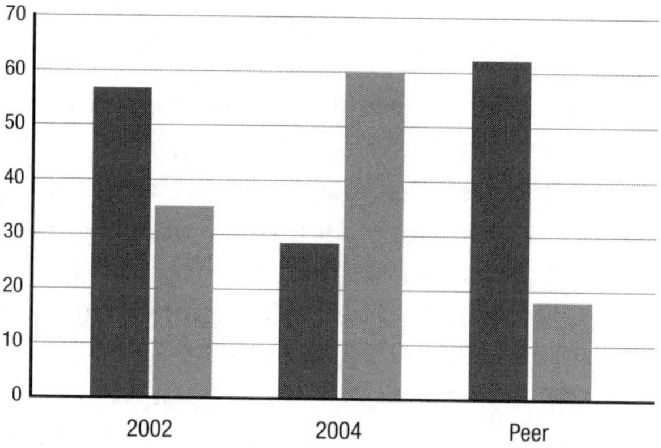

Figure 7-8. Evaluation and management (E&M) coding before and after EMR. More accurate coding with EMRs mean physicians get paid for all they do. Dark bar indicates Level 3 reimbursement; white bar, Level 4.

2. It takes too much time.
   Using the features of the EMR, like electronic messaging and prescription maintenance, Dr. Fera and Dr. Diamond note that they complete 95 percent of their charts during the office visit, and 95 percent of their work by 5 PM. Remote access to the system allows them to finish up from home if they wish.
3. Patients won't like it.
   "Nobody goes to a bank that keeps paper records any more," says Dr. Fera. "Patients are glad that technology is finally catching on in their doctor's office."

Patients appreciate the efficiencies. Their office visits run more smoothly, too, when all lab and pharmacy records are at the doctor's fingertips.

4. Notes are too generic.
"One thing we have learned from other high-risk industries like airlines, is that standardization decreases errors and leads to safer practice," says Dr. Fera.
Electronic medical record notes are in a standardized format, but they are customizable, he points out. The structure leads to discipline, and fewer bits of information are likely to be left out.
5. Staff won't like it.
The staff benefits immediately from certain features of the EMR. E-mail, medlists, and chart-search capabilities, for example, save hours of tedium and boost morale.
"High staff morale translates to high physician morale," says Dr. Fera.
6. It's not secure.
EMR software has the same level of security and encryption as banking software. Charts can be "locked," and the entire system can be audited.
7. It's not stable.
"For physicians concerned about the system crashing, I have only one question: 'How many times were you unable to find a paper chart yesterday?' The paper-based server goes down multiple times per day while our computer server has gone down less than a handful of times over four years," says Dr. Fera.
The EMR system is on constantly, and any maintenance procedures or updates can be scheduled for off-business hours. He reports less technical difficulty and higher reliability with the EMR than with his prior billing/data software.
8. It will take too long to transition into the system.
Some practices opt for a "hard start" on Monday morning with the system and all its features suddenly available. Others prefer to make a more gradual transition, scanning in old paper records as they go. Dr. Fera's practice opted for the gradual transition and

discovered that by the second or third patient visit, paper charts were no longer necessary.

By the way, soon after adopting the EMR, Dr. Fera's practice also improved productivity by adding two new exam rooms.

"They used to be the chart room," he says.

9. It won't improve quality.

The EMR has made it easy for Dr. Fera to track lab numbers of diabetic patients. The ability to do this has produced some significant improvements in the quality of care he is able to provide.

"In our practice, LDL declined, from an average of 110 to 104," said Dr. Fera. "Hemoglobin A1C levels went from 7.8 percent to 7.3 percent. That means that, because of the electronic record, more than seven of 100 diabetics didn't go to the hospital, or lose an eye or a foot."

The practice is currently implementing a patient portal in the EMR, which would allow patients to monitor their lab results and become more active in their own care—a chief tenet of the Wagner Chronic Care Model.

"There is obviously power in biosurveillance as well," says Fera. "There is power in data."

CHAPTER 8

Transforming a Medical Specialty

CASE STUDIES

- **Section 1. Small improvements yield big results in UPMC Shadyside Pathology Lab.** What would it take to apply the principles of Perfecting Patient Care to the numerous, hand-done processes in a pathology laboratory? One hospital's improvement work led to improved turnaround times and improved satisfaction of workers and patients.
- **Section 2. Culture change transforms Henry Ford Hospital Pathology Department.** One physician and one process engineer lead the nation's fifteenth largest pathology unit toward vigorous, rapid-cycle work redesign that is largely employee-driven. The key to all improvements? Culture change.

"Zero defects" is the performance level expected in certain high-risk industries like aviation. In medicine, anesthesiology transformed itself into a specialty striving at all times, for perfect outcomes—a continuous process that entails drilling down into the smallest process defect to eliminate it.

This chapter looks at two pathology departments—one small and one large—that have begun to infuse their work with Toyota-based principles. Using them as a foundation, Henry Ford Hospital has blended the approach with tools borrowed from Six Sigma and other quality improvement initiatives. However, say the Ford team leaders, it was the culture change engendered by the application of the Toyota principles that allowed all other tools to work.

• SECTION 1 •

SMALL IMPROVEMENTS YIELD BIG RESULTS IN UPMC SHADYSIDE PATHOLOGY LAB

Ever wonder what happens to the tissue your doctor sends to the lab? A lot can be riding on the results, and the process may be more complicated than you think. The order resembles an assembly line more than most people would realize. Here's what happens:

Samples first arrive in their complete state in the *Gross Room*, where pathologist assistants perform a gross or "macro" examination of the tissue, dictate notes about its condition, and decide from where to extract the sample(s). After cutting the samples into sections, the tissue is placed into one-inch-square cassettes. The next step is *tissue fixation*, which is the infiltration of the tissue with formalin (a formaldehyde solution). Tissue fixation occurs in a tissue processing machine. Conventional tissue processing can take up to 12 hours.

The samples then arrive in *histology*, where histotechnologists prepare the samples for microscopic examination. The histotechnologists orient the tissue samples in the cassette and embed them with paraffin wax. Once the paraffin is chilled and hardened, the embedded sample is ready to be sliced delicately into super-thin ribbons for application to a slide. The samples then go to another machine for staining.

Only then are the slides ready for the pathologist to review, make a diagnosis, send the results to the patient's physician, and finish the dictation.

Histology: beginning in the middle

Funded by a grant from the Jewish Healthcare Foundation, the Pathology Laboratory at the UPMC Shadyside campus began to experiment with process streamlining in 2004. Project principals include Jennifer Condel, SCT (ASCP) MT, Team Leader; Steven Raab, MD, director, Center for Pathology Quality and Health Care Research, chief of pathology UPMC Shadyside campus; and David Sharbaugh, director of quality improvement.

The basic premise was this: Process time is 24 to 48 hours. That's one or two days for the clinician to wait and the patient to worry. Beginning as usual with the question "Why can't we?" the Shadyside team decided to ask the question this way: *Why can't we get results, at least for the small tissue samples, back to clinicians within 24 hours?*

Because the team planned to use Perfecting Patient Care techniques, and because histology, the midpoint of the work, operated something like an assembly line, the team decided to begin there. Eventually, the goal is to make the entire process—from the Gross Room to the pathologist's interpretation—one continuous flow process.

As Team Leader, Condel's first job was to reassure the histotechnologists. The lab already has a low error rate. "My role was to let them know, 'We aren't changing your work, but with your help, we'll be figuring out how to remove the extra steps and make you even more successful at your job. When you go home for the day, you'll know for sure that the right samples got onto the right slides.'"

As a starting point, several people in the lab took the class offered by PRHI. The discussions and exercises described new ways to look at work, and ways to uncover and resolve problems that were hiding in plain sight—problems that drained the workers' productivity and opened the door to potential error.

Current condition

Before streamlining began, samples stacked up in anticipation of a single 12-hour run in the tissue processor. (This phenomenon, known as "batching," runs contrary to the Toyota principle of doing work one thing at a time, or "one-by-one.") Then the entire batch was fixed in wax, sliced, placed on slides, then stained. There's a paradox in this batching, however. Small tissue samples require only about three hours in the tissue processor, but require more time to embed and cut. Big tissue samples take the full 12 hours in the processor, but less time to embed and cut. Nevertheless, all samples were processed for 12 hours; the batch was run each night; and each morning, processing began en masse.

This batching also extended to the way the samples were prepared from there. Workers would cluster together on each step of the process, creating a crowded, inefficient work space.

Soon histotechnologists discovered some of the inherent problems with batching: "Why should the sample for Patient 1 have to wait for Patient 50's sample to be done before I pass that work down the line?" "Why do I have all these cassettes stacked up when I can only work on one at a time anyway? If I try to work on two at once, I could get them mixed up."

Another problem facing the lab in the beginning was that while they ran short on some materials, others were overstocked and set to expire. It wasn't for lack of effort: The person in charge of ordering expected to spend eight hours a week cataloguing, inventorying, and ordering supplies. Still, people would forget to report a needed item, sometimes resulting in a costly "stat" order. The problem was in the system.

One by one

The group decided to experiment with one-by-one processing. To do so, the lab had to be reconfigured for continuous work flow (Figure 8-1, 8-2, 8-3, 8-4). One evening, a group of hospital and PRHI employees performed a 5S exercise in the lab. It's a disciplined way to clean and organize the workspace (sort, set in order, shine, standardize, and sustain).

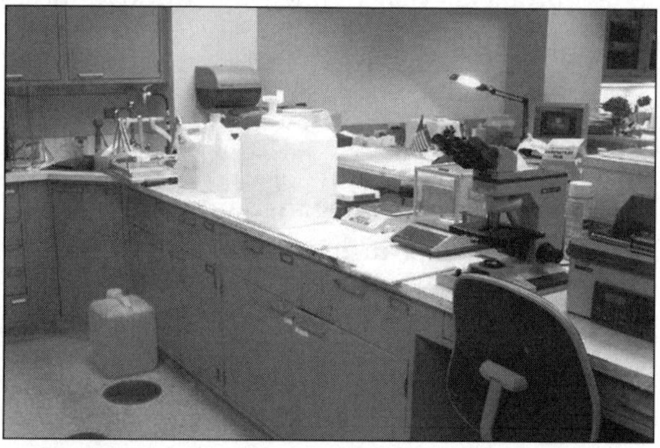

Figure 8-1. *Before*, cluttered workspace that was not set up for continuous work flow.

Once the group members redesigned the workspace, they decided to begin processing the samples one by one. But batching just feels more efficient, and at first, it seemed as if the new one-by-one system lengthened the turnaround time. Technologists began to notice that processing one by one really didn't take any more time, and there was an added bonus: By focusing on one sample at a time, they caught and avoided errors.

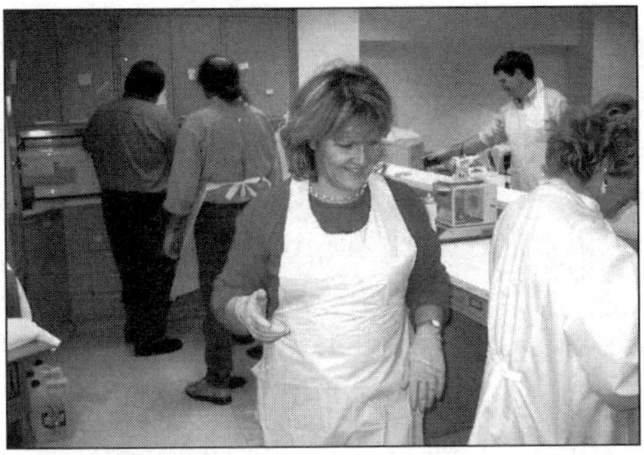

Figure 8-2. Many hands make light work during complete 5S of the pathology lab. Shadyside staff and PRHI staff worked side by side one evening to give the pathology lab a going-over.

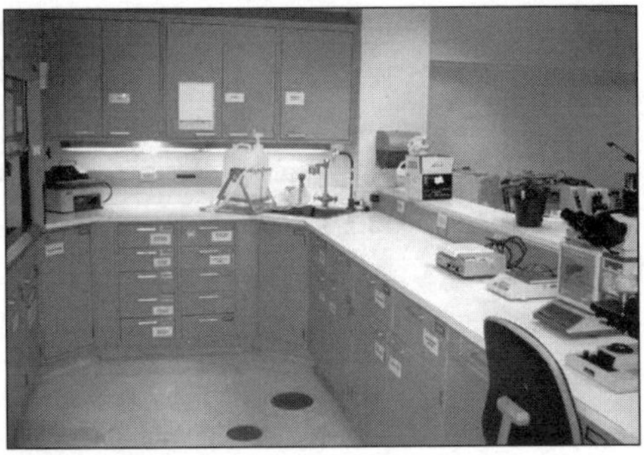

Figure 8-3. Clean lab set up for work flow, right to left around the U-shape.

One problem resulted in a major innovation. Cassettes need to stay cold during processing. Cold trays answered the need when they were batching 10 or 20 samples, but single processing created the need to keep each cassette cold. Histotechnologist Mary Clancy, with help from her father and fiancé, fabricated a device that holds a small block of ice, cooling gel, a space for just one cassette, and a space for the corresponding slide(s). It worked so well that hospital carpenters fabricated 30 more (Figure 8-5).

"I didn't realize we would be so involved in changing our work according to Perfecting Patient Care principles," said Clancy. "This just seemed like we would be told how to do our work, and so I held back.

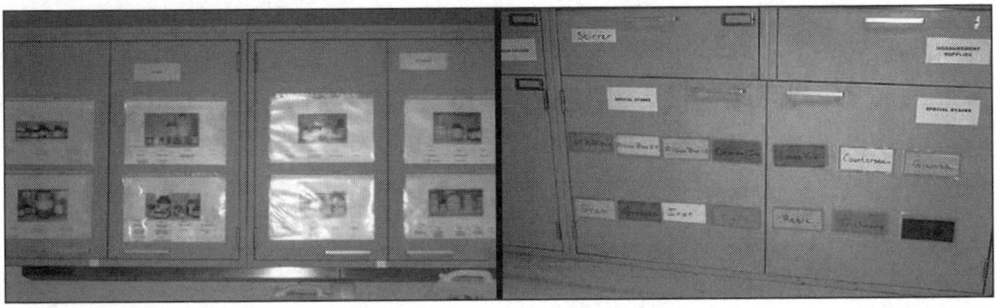

Figure 8-4. With visual cues, there's no doubt about where things are, or where they go. Cupboards are color coded, with contents posted on the outside. The lab, as a whole (and this arrangement in particular) won praise from inspectors from the College of American Pathologists (CAP).

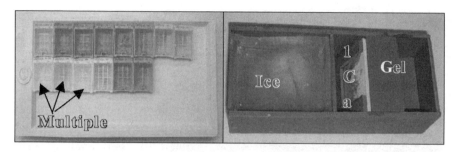

Figure 8-5. Although error rates are extremely low, histotechnologists realized that batching samples (L) opened the door to mistakes. A custom-designed, single-cassette holder (R) keeps discrete cassettes chilled, ready for one-by-one processing.

But we're being told, 'Design your own work, design it from scratch,' and they mean it. It's so liberating!"

The group decided to experiment with the small tissue samples to see if they could reduce turnaround time. Now each morning at 9 AM, a small batch of small tissue specimens run for 3 hours, and specimens are quickly available for reading. What was once a one- or two-day process now has same-day turnaround, and more work can be processed in a day. Furthermore, using the principle of leveling (or equalizing) the workload, the techs now process small and large tissue samples interchangeably, resulting in better flow.

Ordering

Clancy also designed *kanban* cards (Figure 8-6), little inventory cards used as ordering reminders. Almost every item in the lab now has one, so when an item runs low, coworkers put the card on a hook as a visible signal to reorder. Instead of consuming one 8-hour shift, ordering takes just a few minutes per day. Orders are not batched, but take place as needed.

Since the *kanban* system was introduced, stock-outs have been rare, even though inventory has been reduced by 40–50 percent. Costly *stat* shipping has been eliminated, as has been wasted material past its expiration.

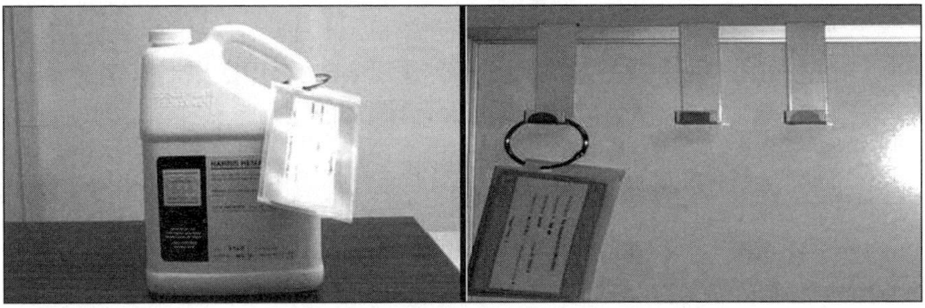

Figure 8-6. When the supply runs low, the kanban card (L) is removed and hung on the ordering hook (R). Ordering is continuous, and takes just minutes instead of one 8-hour work day per week of a professional's time.

Next stop on the line

Pathologist Raab championed the process improvements. Fellow physicians, accustomed to reading large batches of slides, are just beginning to become accustomed to a steady work flow. Dr. Raab is acquainting them with the principle of one by one.

"Eventually we hope to create a continuous-flow, one-by-one processing throughout the whole pathology pathway," says Condel. "It will decrease errors, time, waste, and cost, and make the work more satisfying to the staff."

• SECTION 2 •

CULTURE CHANGE TRANSFORMS HENRY FORD HOSPITAL PATHOLOGY DEPARTMENT

Applying Toyota-based improvements in the pathology department of Detroit's Henry Ford Health System may strike some as ironic. To Richard J. Zarbo, MD, DMD, and certified quality engineer Rita D'Angelo, it merely completes a circle. They insist that lean technology, Six Sigma, and other strategies based on the elimination of waste are not new, and did not originate in Asia. Those ideas stem from Henry Ford's insight that efficiency and productivity arise from the savings produced when waste is eliminated.[1] Ford's insight provided the basis of his 1913 invention, the assembly line, which catapulted Japan's postwar industrial boom into today's manufacturing dominance.

But Zarbo is the first to say that the Toyota Production System and its clinical offshoot, Perfecting Patient Care, are not merely about the relentless elimination of waste. The Toyota approach is about people. It requires nothing less than a complete cultural shift in the American workplace that gives every worker and manager a way to design their work—a blame-free and cooperative work environment—and a way to unleash their profound creative potential.

Zarbo, who holds degrees in both medicine and dentistry, is chair of the department of pathology at Henry Ford Hospital, senior vice president of pathology and laboratory medicine, and program director of Ford's pathology residency program. In March 2007, he was named vice president of the United States and Canadian Academy of Pathology (USCAP).

In the three years since he began to study these industry-based techniques, Zarbo has learned a lot about the nuts and bolts of quality improvement. But he is convinced that the secret of success lies elsewhere.

"For this to work, a top leader—I mean, director level—must be in charge, coaching and coaxing respect and dignity among every person in the organization, and maintaining a focus on the patient," Zarbo said.

1. Keller, Ralph, "Continuous Improvement—Are You Reinventing Wheels?" *Industry Week* (December 1, 2006).

"With a director in charge, people soon realize this is not some new program, but a new way of doing things around here. Having 'no escape' defuses the struggle. I've learned a lot about people since we started—it has to be about them."

Getting started

Intrigued by the work at UPMC Shadyside's pathology department, Zarbo traveled to Pittsburgh for training with PRHI in 2004. The idea was to start with surgical pathology (analysis of tissue) and eventually spread the work to clinical pathology (analysis of blood and urine). Henry Ford Health System's pathology department is the twelfth largest in the country. With 6.8 million blood and urine tests annually, clinical pathology is far larger than surgical pathology. It was decided to start with the smaller side first.

The surgical pathology division typically accessions about 48,000 surgical cases each year. It is staffed by 22 anatomic and surgical pathologists who train 16 pathology residents and two cytopathology fellows.

Zarbo returned from Pittsburgh and trained four others, to see whether or not they thought the approaches could be applied in the pathology environment. Dr. Zarbo tried to implement what he had learned, but the endeavor felt top down and contrived.

Persuading everyone that this would not be the latest "QI thing" proved difficult. Zarbo thought about ways to help the staff start thinking about a more profound transformation. For starters, he believed that the workforce in one of the nation's largest pathology departments needed its own statements of mission, vision and values (Figure 8-7). They also

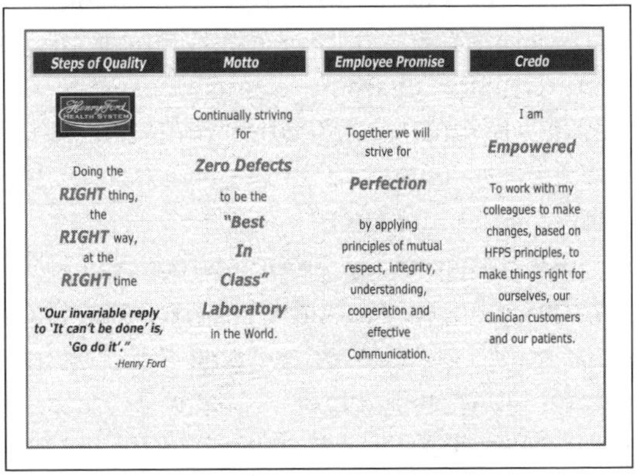

Figure 8-7. Wallet foldout that each employee in the pathology department carries, concerning the mission, vision, and values of the department.

needed a comprehensive approach that borrowed from every successful quality initiative, while remaining rooted in the Toyota principle of a work culture imbued with dignity and respect.

To help devise such an approach, Zarbo hired Rita D'Angelo, a prior laboratory professional who arrived from industry a certified quality engineer and Six Sigma Black Belt and quickly assimilated the principles. The result is called the Henry Ford Production System (HFPS).

Customer–supplier meetings

D'Angelo wasted no time setting up customer–supplier meetings. With a multistep process like preparation of tissue samples in a surgical pathology lab, each worker in the chain takes a turn being a customer (receiving work) and being a supplier (passing it to the next station). But when each step is insulated from the next, suppliers may not know precisely what their customers need. In customer–supplier meetings—kept deliberately brief, out of respect for workers' time—both parties began to describe their needs to one other.

"Usually the response is, 'Oh, I didn't know you needed that! Here, I can do that for you!'" said D'Angelo.

Within nine months, over 100 customer–supplier meetings were held. Customer–supplier teams spring up spontaneously throughout the organization now, and the initiative has extended to the operating room. During the customer supplier meetings, nurse administrators attend by discussing requirements, challenges and constraints in OR and explain how tissue samples originate. Education programs have developed as a result of these meetings to educated staff nurses and lab personnel on how to properly submit and receive OR specimens.

By turns, every employee is expected to present his or her team's improvements at monthly "Share the Gain" meetings. These meetings have transformed over the past three years from tentative, quiet sessions into popular, standing-room-only events, with employees from across the hospital attending.

"Communication went from zero to total," says D'Angelo "We further communicate our changes by the presentation of one process improvement per month, per team, that has developed to be the expectation of all

AP (anatomical pathology) staff. Most important, everyone's work is honored and respected, and that fuels more and more improvement."

Team member Sandra McMahon described the shift in thinking, "Instead of holding tight to how we always did it, we are more aware. These meetings defragment the work and we see where our work fits in."

In the past, the doctor might have been reluctant to mention defects to the technicians, afraid of engendering mistrust or a bad reaction. Now, at weekly group meetings, in the spirit of improving patient care through shared learning, pathologists show the technicians photographs of slides that have given them pause.

"Maybe some samples had been cut a little too thick, or some didn't soak long enough. Something could have been a little clearer. Once we are aware of the problem, we can really reduce the incidence," said McMahon. "Through these meetings, we can see that the quality of slides—the quality of our work—is very important. Now we have good feedback."

"It was unsettling at first, said McMahon of the Henry Ford Production System "You have to get the hang of thinking like this. Now instead of dwelling on every aspect of the problem (including blame), we just start looking for solutions. Everyone here shares a concern about improving quality for patients."

The Share the Gain meetings provide another important incentive.

"We tie rewards to the presentations," said Zarbo. "All employees eventually must present at the quality meetings. It's an important way for everyone to be able to see the problem, and you have to see it before you can start to fix it."

Train them all, train them quickly

D'Angelo began creating educational modules specific to the environment of the pathology lab. She began with 5S training (sort, set in order, shine, standardize, and sustain), assigning specialists for *kanban*, taggers, labelers, stockroom people, cleaners, organizers, and a moving crew (Figures 8-8, 8-9).

Over two months, D'Angelo trained everyone in surgical pathology in modules of one hour over two to three days. To do it, she trained over 200 people in three labs over three shifts. Class size ranged from a minimum of three to four to a maximum of 20. Why?

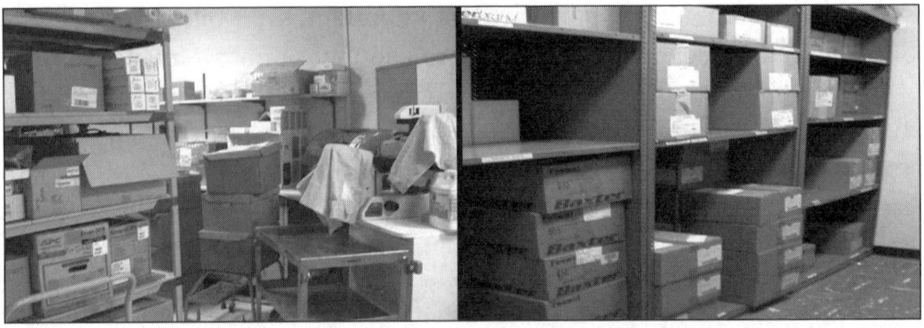

Figure 8-8. 5S *Before* (left) and *After* (right) at Henry Ford Hospital. Training took weeks and required specialization of tasks. The result was less inventory, fewer stock-outs, and less wasted time hunting for supplies.

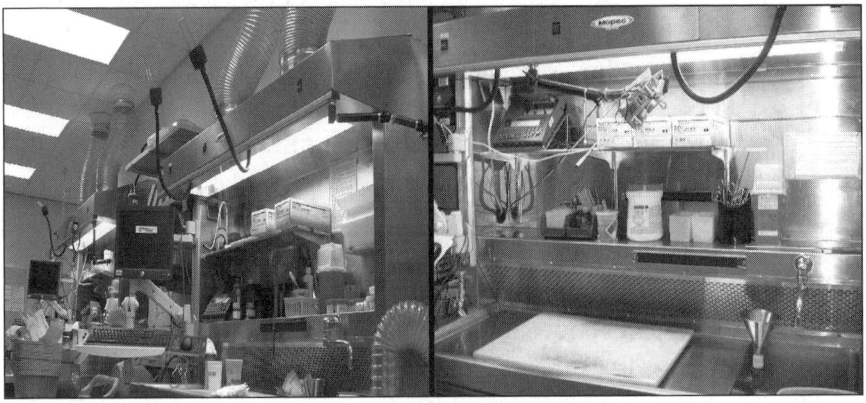

Figure 8-9. 5S used to standardize cutting stations. *Before*, left. *After*, right.

"Training a select few doesn't work," said D'Angelo. "You have to train everybody. And the training works much better in smaller groups. There's more give and take, and people achieve a better understanding."

Training continued on standardized work. This became an in-depth, two-part module tailored to the surgical pathology process. D'Angelo followed each person, mapped each process, reached consensus, standardized, and refined as needed.[2]

2. R. J. Zarbo and R. D'Angelo, "Transforming to a Quality Culture: The Henry Ford Production System," *Am J Clin Pathol*, 126[Supl1]:S21–S29, American Society for Clinical Pathology (2006).

As practiced in Pittsburgh, Perfecting Patient Care training takes four days, but pathology technicians can't be away from their work for more than an hour at any time. Zarbo challenged D'Angelo to convey the Toyota-based concepts as thoroughly and quickly as possible, in the context of work. Exercises that demonstrate concepts like pull (waiting until something is needed before it's produced), continuous flow (keeping the work moving), stores (the few extra to handle extraordinary demand), standardization (reducing variation), communication and leveling (equalizing the work among workers) now take just 55 minutes.

For Zarbo and D'Angelo, one of the most rewarding and exciting parts of the work has been watching the new leaders emerge. Once team leaders were selected, they were put in charge of driving improvement, improving communication, and helping everyone refine processes in the course of work.

Views from the shop floor

Before 5S, before the big changes, there were the pink buckets (Figure 8-10).

"We used them for just about everything," said Connie Shepherd, 10-year veteran surgical pathology technician. She points to a shelf along a wall and says the pink buckets used to line it.

Now, partitioned blue trays provide a way to verify the slide, case information, and the lab tag and provide an instant quality check (Figure 8-11). The cassettes and accessioning information are always together in one cell. Shepherd notes that the technicians devised the idea themselves, and it has allowed them to catch up with the workflow.

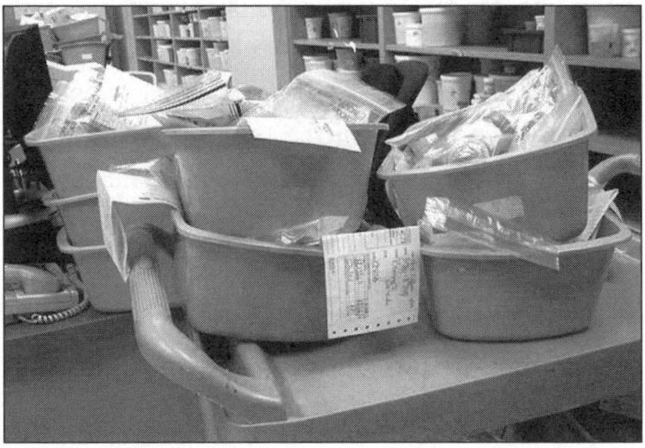

Figure 8-10. *Before*: Samples arrived in plastic bags in pink buckets.

Barbara Dionsi, a 12-year pathology technician, said, "We would never get done. We

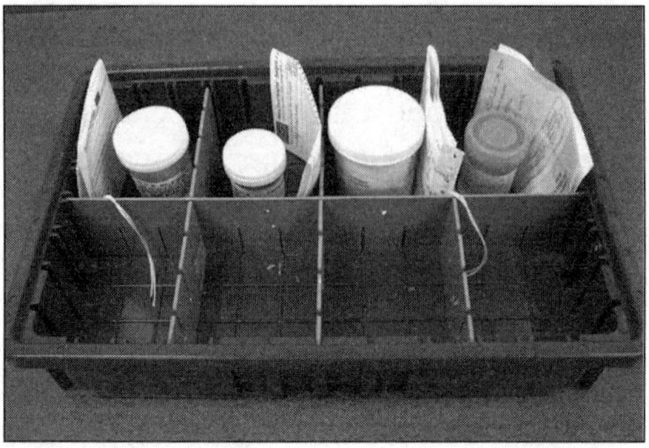

Figure 8-11. *After*: Techs devised divided trays, so paperwork and samples for each patient stay together. The result of standardization has been a 60 percent time reduction in this part of the processing.

were always overwhelmed, stressed, and a day behind. Always."

Still, when Dr. Zarbo and Rita D'Angelo offered a new way to work, Dionsi didn't want to make changes.

"The first week I was really bugged about the changes," she concedes. "By the second week, I started getting it, and by the third week I was suggesting improvements myself."

Today, Dionsi looks forward to coming to work.

"The monotony is broken," she says. "We come up with ideas. We try them. There's no big excitement if something doesn't work; we just try something else. There's an openness that wasn't here before. We have customer–supplier meetings, so we know where our stuff goes after here. That was a revelation!"

Now in the second year, Quality Research Coordinator Ruan Varney maintains those customer-supplier meetings, offering conflict resolution when necessary. Dozens of ideas generated by the workers have taken hold. For example, workers start at 4:30 AM, which is earlier than before. Now slides get out earlier. The processor tray can hold 40 samples, and technicians used to wait until the batch was full to run the processor. Switching to a pull system for the processor, batches are run every 20 minutes regardless of size and a timer is set to sound when it's time to load the processor. The workflow is standardized, and results get out more quickly.

Molecular profile results spur investment, education

Over the past five years, Zarbo and Mark Tuthill, his pathology informatics division head, have spearheaded the development of a surgical pathology barcode system like no other. Not only does it positively identify the patient, but it tells each person what the next process step in production is, which reduces the possibility of defects being passed along and proliferating in the system. The technology is being rolled out in the surgical pathology department. By 2009, an expanded version of this barcode system will go system wide, identifying the collector of the sample as well as the patient. The improvement is based on the principle of "one by one." Patients will be identified at the bedside, and the precise number of correct labels will be printed for test tubes at the bedside.

Other important pieces of technology are a laser etcher that embeds identification information on each tissue cassette and specially developed slide labels so that identifying information cannot be removed by processing chemicals such as xylene. This eliminates hand writing on cassettes and slides, which can introduce defects into the system. Ford was the beta-test site for the technology.

"We ruined a lot of labels along the way," says Zarbo.

Zarbo recognizes that adoption of these new technologies is greatly enhanced by the new culture. "It goes hand in hand," he said. "Toyota prepares the culture ready to accept something big and new, but the electronic system is a huge improvement."

These technologies come at a price—about $6.2 million, to be exact. To maintain momentum for these advances, Zarbo leverages the data. One tenet of Toyota-based improvement relies on describing, as accurately as possible, the current condition. How were patients being identified at the point of collection of their blood samples? What was the rate of correct identification? Zarbo knew that describing the current condition scientifically would entail some laboratory detective work.

To conduct a study using molecular profiling to analyze previous hematology specimens taken on the same patient, he turned to Milena Cankovic, PhD, technical director of Henry Ford's Molecular Pathology Department. The study used complete blood count, or CBC specimens, because it is a routine blood test. Occasionally, the lab will flag a CBC result because it is inconsistent with the result of a recent test on that same patient. Usually, the test is repeated under the general belief that a mislabeling may have occurred by the clinician, nurse, clerk or possibly the laboratory input incorrect information into the database.

In one 6-day period, of 4,269 CBCs processed, the Molecular Pathology Department tested 92 specimens that had been flagged. The positive news was that, of those thousands of tests, the accuracy rate was 99.9 percent. The unfortunate news was that, 0.1 percent of all CBCs processed—three out of those 92 specimens—contained a "discrepant genotype." That is, the specimen belonged to another patient—a misidentification had occurred before the sample had arrived in the lab.

"The hematology and molecular pathology departments quickly summarized results and presented them to a meeting of the Henry Ford Production System," said Cankovic. "Together they devised immediate improvements and strategies for additional training of all personnel who collect specimens."

Zarbo presented the result to the hospital's executive committee, who agreed with him that 99.9 percent accuracy was not good enough. He leveraged the results into increased financial support for his department's work, and a sense of urgency for the new proposed barcode specimen collection and labeling technology.

Education Coordinator Anjna Gandhi immediately began creating education and standardization modules for phlebotomy. At Henry Ford, to foster hands-on care, nurses collect blood samples instead of phlebotomists, who specialize in blood draws. With help from the chief nursing officer and clinical laboratory staff, the pathology department completely standardized the blood-draw process and educated every person who draws blood. Now there is a mandatory online education module, plus mandatory yearly competency testing.

Said Gandhi, "The lab owns the competency training. It's our way of standardizing our suppliers. They've thanked us repeatedly for the module."

The importance of data[3]

Tracking quality data in the discipline of pathology is usually accomplished through subscription quality indicator programs that measure lab

3. R. D'Angelo and R. J. Zarbo, "The Henry Ford Production System: Measures of Process Defects and Waste in Surgical Pathology as a Basis for Quality Improvement Initiatives," *Am J Clin Path*, in press 2007.

data retrospectively for purposes of benchmarking. But no data-gathering device existed that would tell the team, in real time, when a defect in any one process occurred. Generally, a problem is caught at the next process and sent back. Gathering data at the point of origin, before a defect is passed along in the process, was the ultimate goal. First of all, the teams needed to know the current condition—how often were process defects occurring?

To find out, Zarbo, D'Angelo, and team devised a low-tech data-gathering technique borrowed from the Toyota shop floor. The "Andon board" in a factory is an automated system whereby any worker encountering the smallest problem can pull a cord and light a light on the master board, which is visible by all workers. When a problem is tallied this way, in real time, help can be sent, and the real root cause of the problem can more easily be determined. The farther away in time and place the actual problem, the more information is lost. Retrospective data is of limited use.

In surgical pathology, the team surveyed workers to determine the top sources of waste, defect, or misidentification they encountered in the course of their work, and created 100 indicators of these problems. After several tries, they created a data collection tool that caught standardized data in real time, was easy to use and accessible by all employees, and promoted team spirit in a blameless culture—and was reusable. They created laminated posters to capture the information, and provided dry-erase pens for workers to document which problem they had, and how often. Employees were trained, and they gathered data for two weeks in early 2006.

The results were surprising. Of the 1,690 cases tallied, 27.9 percent encountered process defects, most of which arose in the laboratory. Each defect introduced the possibility of rework and waste that could affect the turn around time of patient test results. D'Angelo and Zarbo calculated that, annually, the time spent on rework to correct identification defects alone in AP amounted to 1.3 full-time employees.

Not only did this information help pinpoint where defects were introduced, but because a proportion of the defects involved misidentification, Zarbo used the data to strengthen his case for automation and barcoding.

Data-collection posters continue to be placed in various areas of surgical pathology to measure defects and the effects of the improvement work. In the ensuing year, the defect rate has plummeted from 27.9 percent to 12 percent—a 55 percent decline in waste.[4]

Resident proposes investment in patient safety

The Faxitron imaging machine has been in use in the surgical pathology department for just a few weeks as of this writing. Surgical Pathology Resident Leo Niemeier, MD, whose interest is breast pathology, used data to persuade Zarbo to invest in the expensive digital Faxitron scanner to look for calcifications in breast biopsies. Microcalcifications can be a sign of precancerous changes in the breast.

Niemeier showed that wait time, an average of 3.5 days for breast biopsies, is nerve-wracking for patients and expensive for the system and that histology has to cut twice as many samples—most of it waste—trying to zero in on the calcified areas. Time and materials of the technician and pathologist were wasted. Breast needle biopsies were taken to radiology where delays were common.

With a digital, self-contained Faxitron machine in the pathology department, Niemeier reasoned, pathologists could more quickly focus in on suspect areas without resorting to cumbersome X-rays—old technology that presented problems of film and chemical storage. Technicians would cut fewer blocks and create fewer slides.

"We get the sample the day after surgery. From the point of view of the woman, then, we're already a day behind," said Niemeier. "If we send it to radiology, that brings us to three days to find the target. It's only a handful of cases, but faster, better imaging could make a huge difference."

Using the Faxitron to image the sample allows pathologists to pinpoint the location of the tumor immediately. If the surgery is a lumpectomy with a positive margin, pathologists can reimage subsequent excisions. In a mastectomy and axillary lymph-node biopsy, use of the Faxitron results in better staging for patients.

---

4. R. J. Zarbo and R. D'Angelo, "The Henry Ford Production System: Effective Reduction of Process Defects and Waste in Surgical Pathology," *Am J Clin Path*, anticipated publication 2007.

"It isn't just the financial investment: our quality of pathology and dedication to patients factor in, too," says Niemeier. "Compounded over 12 months in a facility of this size, this 'handful of cases' is actually quite a number." He adds that he found a radiological billing code to ensure that the department is properly reimbursed for use of the Faxitron.

Niemeier noted that the emphasis on the standardization of the workflow in surgical pathology, which had already led to measurable improvements (Figure 8-12) puts the Faxitron in a perfect setting for optimal use.

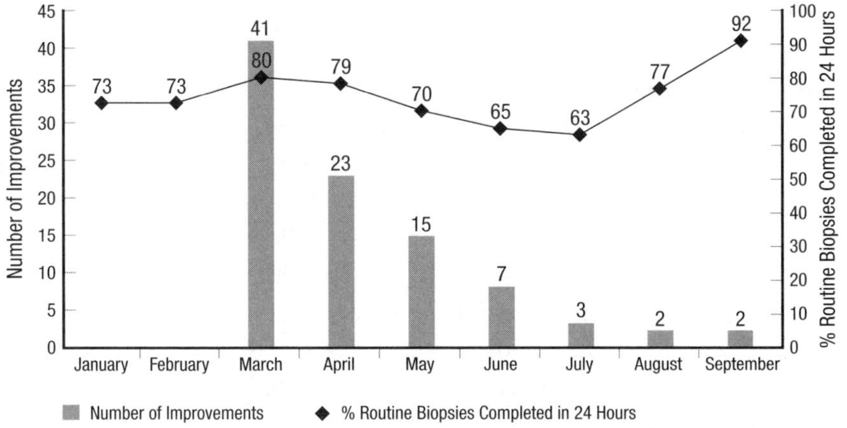

Figure 8-12. Process improvements already led to reduction in turnaround time on breast biopsies. Introducing the high-tech Faxitron machine in an environment of relentless improvement is optimal.

Better processing for prostates

One thing the customer–supplier meetings have made crystal clear: What you do matters for those who work in the process just ahead and behind you. For example, it matters to Pathologist Assistant Nelson Main how specimens are delivered to him in the frozen section lab.

Before, there was no commonly understood standard for delivery, so specimens came in dark plastic bags, or in containers, or containers inside dark plastic bags. Once the upstream suppliers understood that it mattered to Main and his colleagues how the specimens were delivered, those suppliers standardized their work: Specimens now come in clear containers inside clear bags. The intake person marks them off in color-coded pen as they come in to prevent any potential confusion.

But Main was also a supplier. In the case of surgically removed prostate glands, generally enlarged, they are placed in tissue-preserving formalin solution in a container. But while the outer surface of the prostate was preserved, the interior of the gland, which did not contact the formalin solution, tended to degenerate before it got to the cutting station.

Laboratory Technician Vernette Byron said that the cutting of the imperfectly preserved prostates was difficult, often requiring recutting, cutting of more samples than usual, and so forth, to ensure that the pathologist had an adequate sample to read.

"There had been lots of rework," she said.

Main and his colleagues read about a technique of injecting formalin into the gland, completely preserving all of the tissue. After some self-designed experimentation, Main and his colleagues began injecting prostates with formalin solution with great success. The effect for his customer, Byron, and the other technicians, was notable.

"The new process has made all the difference. Now we can embed and cut on the same day, with no waste and no rework," said Byron.

"Patients used to have to wait a week for results," said Main. "Now it's a max of four days. Hospitalization following a prostatectomy usually lasts five days, so the bottom line for the patient is that his results are known by the time he leaves the hospital."

Main looks forward to the new barcoding system, which will generate a xylene-resistant slide label from information entered into the computer system at the time of accession. He calls the technology a breakthrough.

But the real breakthrough, he says, is the deeper understanding that pathology is a process that connects and aligns all work, and all workers.

"I'm from the old school, so at first it was hard," said Main. "You have to change the way you think. Dr. Zarbo taught me you can't be complacent and be competitive. I decided I couldn't live with complacency."

A place for policies

Gandhi notes that the Toyota-based process improvements are not intended to expose defects as much as to standardize internal processes and extend them to external ones.

"The approach is very important," she says. "It's more about awareness and communication. Most people are appreciative. It becomes a better way for us to meet or exceed the national standards."

As part of standardizing external processes, lab personnel are careful to document all defects in process that create delays—whether they originate within or outside of the department. It's no mystery that pathology makes the most entries on the system-wide reporting software, RadicaLogic: The new way of work calls for them to report as many problems as possible, in the interest of learning from and correcting them.

But Henry Ford Health System encompasses 24 outpatient medical centers and numerous clinics in addition to the main hospital. Educating everyone in the vast system on proper sample collection, submittal, and paperwork procedures is Gandhi's daunting task. She notes that a place for well-designed policies issued from top leadership indeed exists. For example:

- The 2001 Specimen Labeling and Acceptability Policy said that any sample that was mislabeled or discrepant in critical-patient and sample identifiers would be rejected. The physician is called. If it's a blood sample, it is discarded, and a new one must be redrawn. If it's tissue, an irreplaceable sample, the ordering physician may rehabilitate it according to a strict process, and must accept responsibility for reidentification of the specimen in writing. Within months of the passage of this policy, there was a 98 percent reduction in defective samples—from 1,769 to 30 defects. Now these defects are rare.
- In 2007, the Specimens Unsuitable for Analysis Policy became instated, which declared that samples could be rejected based on their adequacy for laboratory testing to obtain a meaningful result. For example, if hemolysis was excessive, that is if there was free hemoglobin from lysed red blood cells in the serum of a blood sample, it would be rejected.

- In 2006, nurses were trained in standardized inpatient phlebotomy. In 2007, nurses in outpatient settings were similarly trained.

"A lot of this stuff comes from Henry Ford in 1925," she said. "He said, 'We never fail to make a change once it is demonstrated that the new way is better than the old way.'"

Results

- Same-day turnaround times for routine biopsies improved from 73 percent in January to 92 percent in September. Further improvement for breast biopsies is anticipated with the introduction of Faxitron technology.
- Over the past two years, the surgical pathology lab has seen a 100 percent increase in its workload of genitourinary cases with zero increase in staff.
- Turnaround times for prostate biopsies improved 57 percent, from an average of seven days to four.
- Data at the beginning of the project indicated that work had to be stopped or reworked due to defects in the process about 30 percent of the time. Current data show rework has decreased to approximately 12 percent of the time—a 55 percent waste reduction (Table 8-1).
- In 2006, an internal employee satisfaction survey of laboratory personnel at the Henry Ford Health System rated the pathology department as having the highest focus on quality performance in the system.

Broadening the work

Thus far, the bulk of the process work has been done in Anatomical, or Surgical, Pathology. Zarbo and D'Angelo now seek to broaden the effort into the large and complicated arena of Clinical Pathology.

To kick off the effort Zarbo brought Ford's Clinical Pathology leaders to Pittsburgh for Perfecting Patient Care training in 2007, as he had done for the Surgical Pathology group in 2006, and other leaders in 2005. Over

Table 8-1. Reduction of Surgical Pathology Defect Frequency After One Year of Process Improvements in the Henry Ford Production System.[5]

	Early 2006	Late 2006–Early 2007
Surgical Pathology Cases in Measurement Interval	1,690	1,791
Cases with Defects	472	223
Total Defects	494	288
Defective Case Frequency	27.9 percent	12.5 percent
Proportion of Defective Cases	1 of 3	1 of 8

these three years, PRHI's Perfecting Patient Care curriculum itself had undergone several dramatic improvements, under the leadership of PRHI's Learning Center Staff: Mimi Falbo, MSN, RN; Barbara Jennion, MA; and Tania Lyon, PhD. The training grew shorter, more concentrated, and more closely focused on healthcare. As the groups from Detroit discovered, this training provided a fundamental grounding in how to take the work redesign principles "live" into the workplace.

Zarbo and D'Angelo know the daunting odds facing them, and that 12-hour days and sleepless nights await conscientious leaders trying to implement these principles. That's why Zarbo believes that rapid-cycle improvement must have a director-level person driving it. He doesn't believe that the pathology work at Ford is self sustaining—yet:

"If I went away tomorrow, people would remember this work fondly," he said. "It takes years for the work to become truly enculturated."

He will soon present his findings to the Henry Ford System Leadership Group and Quality Committee of the Board of Trustees. Should Zarbo and D'Angelo's enthusiasm prompt these leaders to embrace interest in taking these principles "wall to wall." Ford would be among the first U.S. hospitals to implement such an ambitious rollout. It would come with some significant up-front costs. But the promise of improved processes is

5. R. D'Angelo and R. J. Zarbo, "The Henry Ford Production System: Measures of Process Defects and Waste in Surgical Pathology as a Basis for Quality Improvement Initiatives," *Am J Clin Path*, in press 2007.

better for patients and workers, and holds the promise of enormous cost saving in the long run.

For those planning to implement a Toyota-based process improvement system, Zarbo advises being prepared for the unexpected.

"This work makes you question everything you've done, and when you do that, you may not know where it will go," he said. "If you are uncomfortable with change, if you don't have self-confidence in your ability to lead, you won't proceed. You have to tolerate insecurity, and never sway in your direction."

GLOSSARY

A-3	A tool of the Toyota Production System and Perfecting Patient Care. Named for the size of 11″ × 17″ paper, A-3s are segmented into quadrants to help teams: 1) map out problems as they exist; 2) define what the ideal situation would look like; 3) hypothesize how to get from here to there; and 4) build in tests.
ACC	Ambulatory Care Center
AGH	Allegheny General Hospital, a hospital within the West Penn Allegheny Health System.
ASC	Ambulatory Surgery Center
BCMA	Barcode medication administration, an electronic barcode reader that helps ensure that the right medication gets to the right patient.
BG	Blood glucose level
CABG	Coronary artery bypass graft surgery. About 350,000 are performed each year in the United States. During CABG surgery, arteries and/or veins are harvested from the body (e.g., from the upper chest or legs) and grafted to the heart to create new routes around narrowed and blocked arteries. This allows enough blood flow to deliver oxygen and nutrients to the heart muscles.
CAP	College of American Pathologists
CCU	Coronary care unit, the intensive care unit for heart patients
CDC	Centers for Disease Control and Prevention, located in Atlanta, Georgia. (www.cdc.gov)
CDU	Child Development Unit at Children's Hospital of UPMC
Chronic Care Model	A model of diabetes care developed by Ed Wagner, MD, of the Seattle-based MacColl Institute.

	(www.researchchannel.org/prog/displayevent.aspx?rID=3877)
CLAB	Central line-associated bloodstream infection, a hospital-acquired infection.
Clostridium difficile (*C.difficile*)	A normal intestinal bacteria, *clostridium difficile* can grow to unhealthy proportions in persons taking antibiotics. The result can be colitis, an inflammation of the intestine, which can then be passed from person to person via unwashed hands.
Continuous flow	Each process completes only the piece that the next process needs in a batch size is one. The one-by-one approach is the opposite of batch-and-queue.
CT scan	Computed tomography (CT), originally known as computed axial tomography (CAT scan) uses X-rays to generate a three-dimensional picture of structures inside of the body.
Eclypsis	An electronic medical record system in use at UPMC Intensive Care Units.
ED	Emergency Department
EMR	Electronic medical record
ER	Emergency Room
FQHC	Federally qualified health center. A federal payment option that enables qualified providers in medically underserved areas to receive cost-based Medicare and Medicaid reimbursement.
Gross room	The room in the pathology lab where specimens are received and "grossed," that is, given a visual or macroscopic examination.
Hemoglobin A1C	A blood test that shows the average amount of glucose in the blood over the past three months. The result indicates whether or not the blood sugar level is under control, which is important in the management of diabetes.

HFPS	The Henry Ford Production System, based on Perfecting Patient Care, and borrowing from other industry-based quality improvement methods.
Histotechnologist	Histotechnologists, or histologists, are laboratory personnel who prepare body tissue for microscopic examination.
ICU	Intensive care unit
IV	Intravenous
JCAHO	The Joint Commission (formerly Joint Commission on Accreditation of Healthcare Organizations), a hospital accrediting body (www.jointcommission.org).
JHF	Jewish Healthcare Foundation of Pittsburgh (www.jhf.org)
Kanban	A tool of the Toyota Production System and Perfecting Patient Care. Kanban cards contain all necessary information for reorder: vendor, contact information, amount to order, and so forth. These cards are placed at a "trigger" point in the inventory, when enough product remains for a specified number of days—more than enough time for the stock to be replenished.
LFHC	UPMC St. Margaret Lawrenceville Family Health Clinic (a FQHC).
Lipid levels	Fats in the blood are lipids. They join with protein in the blood to form lipoproteins, which create energy for the cells of the body. There are three kinds of lipoproteins, (also called cholesterol), in the blood: (1) high-density (also called HDL, for short) cholesterol; (2) low-density (also called LDL) cholesterol; and (3) very low-density (VLDL) cholesterol. Medical conditions such as diabetes can cause elevated lipid levels, which in turn can be a factor in heart disease, stroke, circulatory, and kidney problems.

Mediastinitis	A serious sternal wound infection that can occur following cardiac surgery.
MICU	Medical intensive care unit
MRI	Magnetic resonance imaging, a noninvasive method of medical imaging.
MRSA	Methicillin-resistant *Staphylococcus aureus* is a strain of *Staphylococcus aureus* ("staph") that is resistant to most antibiotics in the medical arsenal.
NNIS	National Nosocomial Infections Surveillance System, developed by the CDC in the early 1970s to monitor the incidence of healthcare-acquired (nosocomial) infections. NNIS is the only national system for tracking these infections. More at http://www.cdc.gov/ncidod/dhqp/nnis.html.
Nosocomial	Infections that are acquired in the healthcare setting are called nosocomial infections.
Nurse Navigators	A year-long program offered to nine nurses by the PRHI's parent Jewish Healthcare Foundation and the Robert Wood Johnson Foundation (RWJF); the Nurse Navigator program offered training and mentoring in the principles of Perfecting Patient Care. The employers for the Nurse Navigators were given a stipend to pay for the training time. For one year, these nurses pursued an aspect of quality improvement in which they had a passionate interest.
OR	Operating room
PCP	Primary care physician
Physician Champion	In early 2006, the PRHI partnered the Allegheny County Medical Society and the Pennsylvania Medical Society to inaugurate the Physician Champions program. The Jewish Healthcare Foundation provided $25,000 grants to support each of six clinical projects run by eight physi-

	cians. All Physician Champion teams learn the principles of Perfecting Patient Care through PRHI's Four-day University and receive on-site coaching from PRHI staff members.
PPE	Personal protective equipment, such as gloves, gowns, and caps, used by healthcare personnel when caring for a patient with a contagious condition.
PRHI	Pittsburgh Regional Health Initiative (www.prhi.org)
Push and pull	In a "push" system the product is produced without consumer request. In a "pull" system it's the consumer's request the "pulls" the product through manufacture and delivery. The "pull" practice reduces wasteful stockpiles and makes replenishment easier.
RWJF	Robert Wood Johnson Foundation (www.rwjf.org)
SICU	Surgical intensive care unit
Standardization	Nonstandard processes, those that vary from one time to the next, are chaotic and not measurable. In the Toyota system, processes must be standardized before continuous improvement can occur and be measured.
UPMC	The University of Pittsburgh Medical Center
UTI	Urinary tract infection
VAP	Ventilator-associated pneumonia (a nosocomial infection)
VAPHS	Veterans Administration Pittsburgh Healthcare System
West Penn	The Western Pennsylvania Hospital, a facility within the West Penn Allegheny Health System.
Whys, five	To get to the root of a problem, the teams will first define the problem as specifically as possible. Then, they will ask themselves "Why?" five times as a way to find the precise cause.
WPAHS	West Penn Allegheny Healthcare System

INDEX

ABOUT THE AUTHOR

Naida Grunden has been a business and technical writer for over 25 years, specializing for the past six years in health and medical writing for the Pittsburgh Regional Health Initiative. She writes the *PRHI Executive Summary* newsletter, a publication she founded in 2001 (www.prhi.org). Her work has appeared in publications as varied as the *Joint Commission Journal on Quality and Patient Safety* and *Air Line Pilot* magazine.

Grunden received the 2006 Challenge Award from the American College of Clinical Engineering for her article, "Industrial Techniques Help Reduce Hospital-Acquired Infection," in *Biomedical Instrumentation and Technology* magazine.

Grunden completed her BA in English at California State University, East Bay, and her secondary English teaching credential at California State University, San Francisco. She lives in Bellingham, Washington. Visit her website at www.NaidaGrunden.com.